D0201342

7 —

STAND BY ME

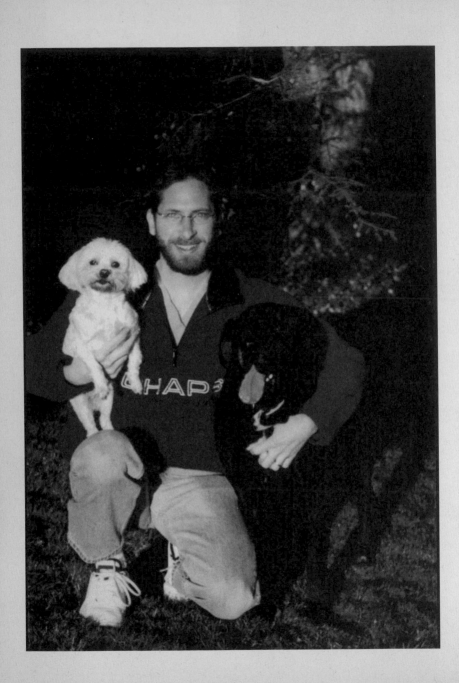

STAND BY ME

A Holistic Handbook

for Animals, Their People, and the Lives They Share Together

WITH WISDOM FROM THE EDGAR CAYCE PHILOSOPHY

By Douglas E. Knueven, D.V.M.

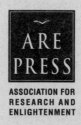

ARE PRESS

ASSOCIATION FOR
RESEARCH AND
ENLIGHTENMENT

A.R.E. Press • Virginia Beach • Virginia

Copyright © 2003
by Douglas E. Knueven, D.V.M.

1st Printing, April 2003

Printed in the U.S.A.

All rights reserved. No part of this book may be reproduced or transmitted in any form or by any means, electronic or mechanical, including photocopying, recording, or by any information storage and retrieval system, without permission in writing from the publisher.

A.R.E. Press
215 67th Street
Virginia Beach, VA 23451–2061

Library of Congress Cataloguing–in–Publication Data
Knueven, Douglas E., 1961–
    Stand by me : a holistic handbook for animals, their people, and the lives they share together / by Douglas E. Knueven.
        p.   cm.
    ISBN 0–87604–440–2 (pbk.)
    1. Pets–Psychic aspects. 2. Pets–Diseases–Alternative treatment. 3. Holistic medicine. 4. Human–animal communication. 5. Cayce, Edgar, 1877–1945. Edgar Cayce readings. I. Title.
SF412.5.K578 2003
636.088'7'019–dc21

                                                    2003000736

Edgar Cayce Readings © 1971, 1993, 1994, 1995, 1996
by the Edgar Cayce Foundation.
All rights reserved.

Cover design by Richard Boyle

Dedication

To my beacon of light, my wife, Judy

Contents

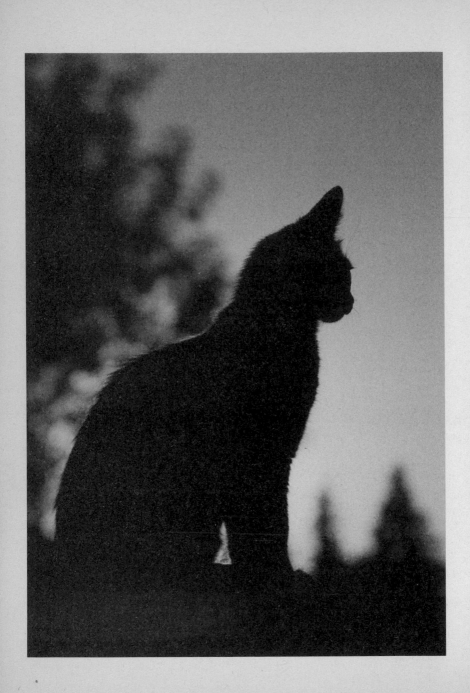

INTRODUCTION

This book is for the true animal lover. For all of us in this growing segment of the human population, our pets are family
members. In fact, the term pet hardly applies. Animal companions or friends are more appropriate terms. We form unbreakable bonds
with our animals that non–animal lovers will never understand.

In my view, any holistic guide for our animal companions must
honor their inner natures as well as their physical structures. The invisible human–animal bond is the most essential facet of the way of life of
both the creature and the person. This is a truly holistic handbook because it gives guidance regarding all aspects of our four-legged friends,
especially the all–important pet connection.

I plan to take you on an exploration of your relationship with your
animal friend. We will start off with a discussion on what it means to
relate with an animal companion. Then, beginning at youth, we will
look at how to choose the perfect companion. We will then discover

methods of communicating with and training your pet. Next we will look at the world of holistic health for animals. We will also investigate the issues of euthanasia, death, and grief. Finally, we'll examine the lessons we all can learn from our furry friends.

My own life's path has led me to an attitude of amazement toward the animal kingdom. Although I was raised in a suburban neighborhood, my parents had roots that deeply tied them to farm life. As a child my daily chores included caring for our pets as well as the rabbits and chickens we raised in the attic of our two-car garage.

Much of my spare time was spent catching snakes, turtles, and the like from the nearby lakes, streams, and woods. Whenever I caught a new creature, I would run to the library and read all about it. I usually kept the critters for the summer, and then returned them to the wild for their winter hibernation. As I look back, I realize I had an uncanny knack for finding and capturing my wild, little friends.

I enjoyed learning at school and had a special love for biology. It was no surprise to my parents when I chose to go to college with my sights set on veterinary school. After a grueling three years in undergraduate school majoring in zoology, I was accepted into the Ohio State College of Veterinary Medicine.

I have to tell you that formal veterinary training is enough to turn a person's love for animals into a relationship with hard, cold facts. We started with such classes as anatomy in which we cut into the dead specimens in an attempt to understand what makes this machine tick. We studied each body system in turn, learning how it worked and how it was affected by disease. It was not until the end of our junior year that we actually got to touch and work with living creatures. Animals were seen as machines and we were the mechanics.

If it were not for my job as an assistant at a local veterinary clinic, I fear my love for animals may have been trained right out of me. My assistant work kept my pet connection alive. I took pleasure in talking to the dogs and cats as I fed and treated them. I also observed the human-animal bond with great interest as I interacted with clients and patients.

I graduated from vet school in 1987 and embarked on my dream career in veterinary medicine. However, within a few years, I began to feel frustrated with the shortcomings of conventional veterinary medicine. Many conditions did not respond to standard treatments. I felt a piece of the puzzle was missing.

About this time, a friend invited me to an "A Search for God" study group. These groups, sponsored by the Association for Research and Enlightenment (the A.R.E.), explore the work of Edgar Cayce—a psychic that is considered by some to be the father of holistic medicine. As the Cayce health philosophy permeated my personal life, I started to look for a way to apply it to my patients.

Castor oil packs, a common Cayce remedy, on an ailing Persian cat sounded mighty messy, and I wasn't quite ready for psychic energy healing. My rational mind needed a more concrete starting point. Being the most researched of the alternative therapies, veterinary acupuncture seemed to be the logical foundation for my understanding of alternative veterinary medicine and the invisible forces that regulate health.

So, my expedition into holistic pet care began in the form of veterinary acupuncture training and practice. Chinese medicine shares many concepts with the Cayce health readings. The idea of a vital energy, which the Chinese call Qi (pronounced *chee*), the complex relationships between the organ systems, and the living consciousness of all tissues of the body were concepts I found familiar after studying the readings.

Since my certification by the International Veterinary Acupuncture Society (IVAS), my eyes have been opened to the merits of other alternative therapies, and my studies and expertise have broadened. But it was really my personal experiences with the animals and their people that moved me to continue pursuing alternative therapies.

Sammy was my first animal teacher in this area. He proudly strolled across my exam table in September of 1994, just before I started my formal acupuncture training. His sleek black coat hid the fact that he was twelve years old and on the verge of the fight of his life.

I soon learned that the inflamed gums that concerned his owner were more than just a simple case of gingivitis. A biopsy revealed squamous cell carcinoma. This aggressive form of cancer does not respond well to chemotherapy, and

Sammy's owners did not want to put him through painful, disfiguring surgery. I prescribed antibiotics and sent him home, instructing his family to keep him comfortable and to bring him back for a humane euthanasia when he stopped eating.

Six weeks later, I returned from the first segment of the IVAS course armed with a handful of small, stainless steel needles and the rudiments of knowledge about Chinese medicine. I called Mary and Ron with new hope for helping their special feline. Acupuncture is not a cure-all, but we all felt we had nothing to lose, so they brought Sammy in for the first of many acupuncture treatments.

His condition had deteriorated considerably since I had last seen him. The left side of his face was severely swollen and a huge crater replaced the inside of his upper jaw. The cancer had spread, and lymph nodes in his neck were so swollen you could see them sticking out through his dull fur. He spent his time at home hiding under the bed, and his appetite had already dropped off. The end seemed near.

Within the first two weeks of acupuncture treatment, the owners noticed improvement. Sammy began eating and playing again. I noticed that the facial swelling was reduced and the hole in his mouth was filling in. I couldn't believe my eyes. I was sure it was the new antibiotic I had put him on that was making the difference. The owners were convinced that the acupuncture was helping, so I continued the treatments.

One day as I was treating Sammy, I mentioned to Mary that I was disappointed that nothing seemed to affect the enlarged lymph nodes. She said that the swelling did subside for a few days right after the acupuncture, but blew up again by the time of his next appointment. That was when I realized that it really was the acupuncture that was helping.

I wish I could say that we cured Sammy's cancer with acupuncture, but we did not. We did, however, buy him a few extra months of quality time with his loving caregivers. I know Sammy and his family truly cherished that extended time to prepare for the inevitable.

In the end, Sammy went downhill quickly. On a cold February morning in 1995, Mary and Ron knew it was time for the final farewell. With tears in my eyes, I gave the injection to end his suffering, and I realized that although I hadn't cured Sammy of cancer, he had cured me of my left-brained skepticism. I would never be the same again.

I have since made it a personal mission to bridge the gap between holistic and conventional medicine, both in the veterinary community and in the general pet–loving population. With every year of practice, I appreciate the bond shared by humankind and our loyal, furry friend more and more. I see the healing effects of companion animals on people, and I stand in awe of the many manifestations of God's love. To me, this feeling is the true meaning of the pet connection.

The journey upon which we are about to embark will be guided not only by myself, but we will also at times be peering through the clair-voyant eyes of Edgar Cayce himself. So our voyage will have a balance of practical experience and mystical insight.

Edgar Cayce was the most documented psychic of the twentieth cen-tury. He dedicated his life to helping others through his extrasensory gift. Mr. Cayce had the ability to put himself into a trance, allowing him to connect with a deep level of consciousness, a dimension of knowing beyond the grasp of most of us. While in this state, he gave discourses, called readings, on subjects including holistic health, spirituality, dreams, meditation, and ancient civilizations, just to name a few. Over 14,000 of these readings were carefully transcribed and meticulously cataloged. Although Edgar Cayce died over fifty years ago, his inspiring message lives on in the work of the A.R.E., the organization he founded to study the material in the readings.

Unfortunately, Edgar Cayce did not have a lot to say about pets spe-cifically. His reply to a distraught pet lover who requested a medical reading for her sick Cocker Spaniel makes his position clear.

> "No, have had many requests for such readings as you asked for—but have never undertaken such; there seems always to be so much to be done to try and help our fel-low man, seem never to have had the time for such. Oh I realize there are many who are just as anxious about their pets as others are about their children but have never been able to persuade myself to undertake such when so many children are so in need, and am very limited even to the number am even able to try and help, tho have been doing

the work for 40 odd years now have not been able to
increase the number can try and help."

Let's face it, Edgar does not fit our definition of an animal lover. Sure, he was fond of all animals, but his priority was the human species.

In Mr. Cayce's defense, we need to realize that he was raised on a farm in the late 1800s. It was a rugged life where animals had their place. This lifestyle required a very utilitarian relationship with the animal kingdom.

Yet, a couple of stories still survive that show a distinctive side to Edgar Cayce's relationship with the animals in his life. The first is an anecdote that appeared in the July 1958 *A.R.E. Bulletin*.

> "Mr. Frank Mitchell, a recent visitor from New York, was a personal friend of Mr. Cayce's. While here, he related an incident of Mr. Cayce's boyhood that has not yet appeared in print:
>
> "As a young boy on a Kentucky farm, Edgar Cayce owned a large dog of uncertain antecedents that was generally classified as a shepherd. (His name was Wallace.) When several sheep were killed by some marauding animal in the neighborhood, Edgar's dog was suspected and accused of the crime. One day a party of farmers arrived with guns to destroy the culprit.
>
> "Neither Edgar nor his great uncle believed the pet was guilty, so they hid it until the farmers went away. As soon as it was released, the dog led the man and boy to a field where some sheep were grazing and lay down in the bushes to wait—Edgar and his uncle doing likewise.
>
> "Presently another large dog slipped out of the brush across the field and, before the watchers could prevent it, attacked and killed one of the sheep. On this eyewitness evidence, provided by the canine detective, the guilty dog was caught and dealt with according to his crimes—and the good reputation of Edgar Cayce's dog was restored."

The second remarkable tale is from Edgar Cayce's 1938 memoirs.

"Among the first jobs given Eddy was to plough a field of corn. A mule and a plow were given him and he was sent to the 100 acres field alone. In the evening when it was getting dark he took out his mules from the plow and mounted, rode to the house. The owner with the other men on the farm were in the lot as he rode up. He noticed all the men looking at him strangely, when the owner rushed out and yelled, 'Get down, get down, that mule will kill you, she has never been ridden before.' But she hadn't shown any signs of disagreement to Eddy's mounting her. But when one of the men on the place attempted to ride her a few days later, she immediately threw him, and was never ridden so far as I know by any one but Eddy that one time, for she was not given to Eddy to plow again. All are still wondering how it was, or why it was she allowed that boy to ride her that evening."

So, the young Edgar did have a unique rapport with animals. And yet, we have to dig deeply into the readings for insights on our relationships with our pets. In spite of the lack of explicit pet information, the readings are rich with wisdom on consciousness, spirituality, holistic living, and our relationship with all of God's creation. From this material we can glean a higher view of the pet connection.

Even though Edgar Cayce himself was not what I would consider a true animal lover, there was one pet that got plenty of attention in the Cayce readings—the little dog Mona.

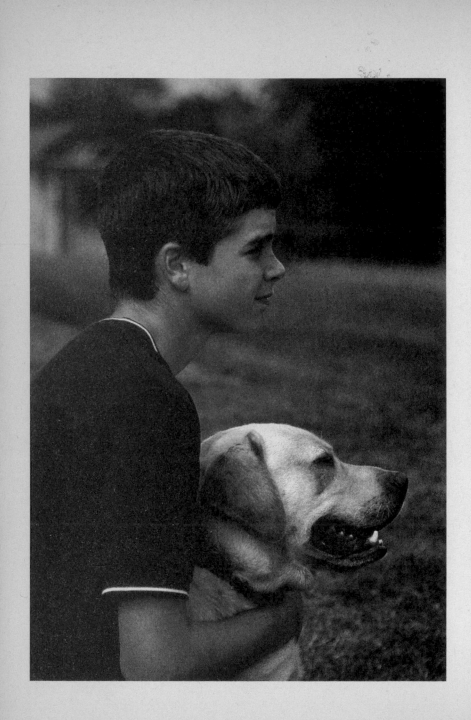

CHAPTER

1

THE PET CONNECTION

(Q) What relation is he to the little dog Mona?
(A) He fought with the body in the Roman experience.
(Q) What was Mona then?
(A) The lioness that fought with the entity . . .

Edgar Cayce Reading 280-1*

T he above reading about a shared past–life experience between man and beast is what inspired this book. What are the implications of the concept of the reincarnation of animals? What other secrets concerning our relationships with our animal friends

---

*In order to preserve anonymity, each Cayce reading recipient has been assigned a numeric reference number instead of the name of the person. In the above reading, 280 refers to the individual, and the number following the dash indicates that this is the individual's first reading.

lay dormant in the Edgar Cayce readings?

As it turns out, the little dog Mona was the most inspiring pet in all of the Cayce readings. Five different individuals requested information about this feisty Pomeranian during their sessions with Edgar. What an awesome creature she must have been to have touched so many lives so deeply. Throughout this book we will investigate other readings regarding Mona in order to learn more about our own human–animal relationships.

Relationship

Before we can investigate how to relate holistically with our animal friends, we need to explore just what is meant by the term relationship. *Webster's New World Dictionary* defines relationship as "the connections between or among persons, nations, etc." So, what is it that connects us with animals? The answer that comes to mind is Life! We share the One Life Force or Spirit.

Having a relationship means sharing Life with another. From the mundane, everyday activities to the sublime moments when everything comes together, we share Life with our animal companions. And they respond. Animal beings provide a level of love for their human friends that is sometimes lacking among people. Interacting with animals appears to be more life-giving to some of us than relating with each other.

Much has been written in the past few years about the magic of the human–companion animal bond. Scientists have even studied the effects of this relationship. A rash of research projects published in the past twenty years have proven the health benefits of sharing Life with companion animals.

In 1980, a study at Brooklyn College found that heart attack victims who own pets live longer than those who do not. A 1992 Australian study revealed that pet owners are less likely than non-pet owners to develop heart disease in the first place. In 1999, research showed that an animal's calming influence worked better to control blood pressure than hypertension medication.

Research with children has shown that pet ownership helps kids learn compassion and responsibility, think more independently, have more self-esteem, and better coping skills, and have less stress, aggression, and sadness. Another study found that having animals in inner-city classrooms dramatically lowered truancy and increased children's test scores. Contact with companion animals has also proven beneficial for children with autism and attention deficit disorder.

Studies of nursing homes in New York, Missouri, and Texas have found amazing benefits of bringing plants and animals into the living quarters. Patient death rates dropped 40 percent and the need for medication was cut in half. University of Nebraska Medical Center researchers demonstrated that pet birds reduced depression and loneliness in elderly people in hospitals and nursing homes.

Several studies have shown that pet owners of all ages had fewer doctor's visits than people without pets. Czech scientists studying the effect of isolation on people say that animals are so essential to human health that they should be included in long-term space flights. It has been proven that people who share their lives with animals live longer than those who do not.

Perhaps the health secret of the human-animal bond lies in the fact our furry friends love us no matter what. They are our best psychotherapists because they are totally nonjudgmental. They simply do not care about our age, social status, or even the way we look. Plus, their therapy fees are comparatively low. Animals have an uncanny knack for sensing our moods and helping us through every crisis. Our creature companions seem to have an innate healing ability.

It appears that sharing Life with an animal enlivens us with a healing presence. The master Jesus promised us that, "For where two or three come together in my name, there am I with them." (Matt 18:20 NIV) This saying troubled me for quite awhile. Why isn't Christ with us when we are alone? Can I not find Him in my meditations? Then I realized that it is through our relationships with others that we truly meet our Maker and join in the Oneness that is God. Our relationships with our animal companions help to fulfill this need for unity. Could it be that as I gaze lovingly at my Maltese DJ, I am looking into the eyes of the Master?

If the concept of seeing the Divine in the eyes of your pet bothers you, consider one of the greatest animal lovers of all time, Saint Francis of Assisi. This gentle soul had a remarkable relationship with the animals he encountered. He reasoned that since the same hand made both them and us, we share a common father. And what do you call someone who has the same father as you? Brother or sister. Francis's famous poem "Canticle to Brother Sun and Sister Moon" is a beautiful celebration of the sacredness of all life, all creation.

According to the Gospel of Mark, the last instruction of Jesus to His apostles was to "preach the gospel to every creature." (Mark 16:15 KJV) Saint Francis took this reading to heart. Francis is said to have reasoned with and even entered into contracts with animals. He once delivered a sermon to a flock of birds. And for their part, the birds attentively listened to the words of the saint. We may never understand what was gained by this exchange, but the story warms the heart of the animal-loving listener.

A Biblical Perspective

Let us look more deeply into the Bible. In the book of Genesis, we find that God's intention when creating the animals was to find a helper for man so he would not be lonely (Gen. 2:18). All creatures were given the same "breath of life" as man (Gen. 6:17). After creating the living creatures God looked at what He had done and "God saw that it was good." (Gen. 1:25)

So good in fact that the creatures were never meant to be killed and eaten by man or even each other.

Then God said [to mankind], "I give you every seed-bear-

ing plant on the face of the whole earth and every tree
that has fruit with seed in it. They will be yours for food.
And to all the beasts of the earth and all the birds of the
air and all the creatures that move on the ground—everything that has the breath of life in it—I give every green
plant for food."   (Gen. 1:29-30 NIV)

God cared so much for all the creatures that Noah was made to go to
great lengths to spare them from the flood. And after the flood had
cleansed the earth, " . . . God remembered Noah and all the wild animals
and the livestock that were with him in the ark . . . " (Gen. 8:1 NIV) God
then set His rainbow in the sky as a sign of His covenant with Noah and
with "all living creatures of every kind." (Gen. 9:15 NIV)

Jesus Himself entered this world among animals in a stable. News of
His birth was first heralded to shepherds—animal caregivers. Jesus often
referred to animals in His stories and likened Himself to the "good shepherd." One of the last public efforts of His life involved freeing the animals that were to be sacrificed at the temple. I think it is safe to say that
Jesus was an animal lover.

It is true that after creating man, God gave him "dominion" over all
the living creatures. But, what does it mean to have dominion over the
animals? One definition of dominion is "power to rule," as a king.

There is no doubt that all creatures, both wild and domestic, are at
the mercy of mankind's dominion. For countless generations, man has
exploited his "power to rule" over the birds of the air and over every
living thing that moves upon the earth. We have ruled many species
into extinction.

But, how is man meant to rule? How does a good king rule? Jesus
told his apostles, "You know that the rulers of the Gentiles lord it over
them, and their high officials exercise authority over them. Not so with
you." (Matt 20:25,26 NIV) Just like the good shepherd, a good ruler serves
his subjects. We are meant to live in harmony with our animal brothers
and sisters, making decisions with their interests in mind. With such a
loving intention perhaps we can relate to our pets, not just physically,
but at the soul level.

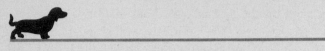

Do Animals Have Souls?

On the physical level, we have quite a lot in common with our pets. Our body structures are very similar. We share many of the same diseases, such as stomach ulcers, diabetes, cancer, arthritis, and glaucoma, just to name a few. Recent scientific studies have shown that even our DNA is 98 percent identical to that of certain primates. So, just what differentiates us from our fellow passengers on planet Earth? Are our pets simply hairy little people walking around on all fours?

In order to truly relate with our companion animals, it is necessary for us to appreciate their deeper aspects. Many of us have such an understanding on an intuitive level. I hope to open your mind further to the possibilities of the hidden facets of animal beings and the implications of considering this deeper level.

As I previously mentioned, Edgar Cayce did not directly address many of the issues we are about to explore. What we learn from the readings on the subject of the nonphysical aspects of animals will require some reasoning and extrapolation on our part. In the end, we may have dug up more questions than answers. There is certainly value just in raising such issues. Ultimately, we must each answer these queries for ourselves. We learn as much about ourselves as we do our animal companions when we delve into these phenomena.

Dreamy Creatures

Most animal lovers have witnessed what looks like dreaming in their pets. The animal's legs move as if they are running. Sometimes my own dog gives out a shrill yip as if he has been attacked. Many pets seem to be quite active during sleep, just as we are when we have a vivid dream.

Research indicates that we dream during specific periods of sleep termed REM sleep. The dream phase was given this name to denote that it is accompanied by rapid eye movement under the closed eyelids. REM sleep is also associated with particular brain waves as detected on electroencephalograms (EEGs).

It is interesting to note that our pets also have periods of rapid eye movement. Scientists have discovered that this animal REM sleep is accompanied by the same brain wave pattern as our REM sleep is. In fact, investigators who specialize in sleep study often use animals hooked up to the EEG to explore various aspects of sleep.

The similarity of animal's REM sleep to ours, coupled with their un-mistakable dream activity, leaves no doubt that animals dream. And, imagine the implications of that statement. We are still exploring the ramifications of our own dreams. One important question is, "Why do we dream?"

Edgar Cayce had much to say about the importance of dreams. He gave several purposes for dreams including giving insight into our daily lives and our higher levels of consciousness.

Dreams as are presented to the body are for the enlight-enment of the consciousness of the body, would the body apply same in the life.   3937-1

From the Cayce perspective, nothing important happens to an individual that has not been foretold in a dream.

Psychologists and psychiatrists since the days of Freud have used dreams to unlock the deep unconscious mental issues of their patients. Thomas Edison used his dreams to solve the problems he ran into as he created new inventions. Elias Howe's dreams inspired him in his invention of the sewing machine. Robert Louis Stevenson was moved creatively by his dreams. In fact, the entire plot for "Dr. Jekyll and Mr. Hyde" came from a dream, as did many of his stories. Great composers such as Richard Wagner and Handel attribute their works to their dreams.

Both the Old and New Testaments of the Bible are full of stories of God sending messengers to mankind through his dreams. Think of the story of Joseph who interpreted Pharaoh's dream. There are also many dreams involved in the Christmas story. Both Joseph and the wise men were given guidance from their nocturnal visions.

As we become aware of the significance of our own dreams, the question arises, "What is the purpose of our pets' dreams?" Do pets have deep psychological issues to work through? Are they inventing new ways of getting into the garbage? Or, perhaps God himself is whispering into their furry ears. And, if like us they dream, might animals also share other "human" qualities?

Beastly Emotions

Emotions are reactions of the body to the perception of inner and outer events. In fact, the root word for the word "emotions" means *to move.* They are the motivating influence in life. The Cayce readings claim that our emotional character is stored in the soul and manifests as bodily responses through the action of the endocrine system.

Emotions are what make us who we are. Some people think that emotions are uniquely human attributes. Everyone knows that animals are biological machines driven only by instinct and hormones, right? That's what I was taught about animals in veterinary school. But, we animal lovers know better.

My personal experiences with animals, as well as the experiences of the countless pet owners I have come to know in my fifteen years of practice, lead me to believe that animals are capable of a full range of emotions. Pets sure seem happy when we put the food bowl down in front of them. They also seem to enjoy play, just for the fun of it. Besides, hasn't your animal companion ever pouted when he didn't get his way? I've been given the "cold shoulder" by many a patient who disapproved of my interference in his day. I've also treated animals that were sick with grief over the loss of a loved one. Most animal lovers have had the experience of being comforted by a pet. Some dogs that I have known even seem proud of their new look after being groomed. They carry themselves differently.

But, maybe all this talk is just anthropomorphism. Humans seem to project their own characteristics on everything. Instead of the imaginary friends we have in childhood, we create animal friends.

On the other hand, even the scientifically minded realize that animals experience the emotion of fear. Of course, scientifically, animal fear is a behavior based solely on the fight or flight response governed by the adrenals. It is strictly an instinct that keeps animals out of the way of danger. But then, what about human fear? Is what we experience as fear any different than what animals feel? The only difference I see is that mankind has perfected fear. We have developed a plethora of anxiety disorders enough to keep the shrinks and pharmaceutical companies in business for years.

But wait! Our animal friends are not to be outdone. What about separation anxiety, the fear-driven destructive behavior that some overly dependent dogs exhibit when left alone in the house? How can this be considered a manifestation of instinct? And, did you know that some animals suffer from obsessive-compulsive disorder? Conventional veterinarians use the same drugs that medical doctors use to treat humans for this condition.

Animals seem to suffer from a lot of the same emotional problems that people do. In fact, animals often mirror their owner's emotional conditions—or is it vice versa? It is certainly true that the number of animal psychological disorders have increased in direct proportion to the incidence of human emotional instability. I think this is more than coincidence.

If animals have emotions, is this evidence of their soul nature? What implications does this notion have on how we treat and interact with our companion animals?

Animal Intuition

Over the years, I have heard a lot of stories of what seems to be psychic pet behavior. At first I figured that some pet owners exaggerate the deeds of their pets. On the other hand, perhaps the strange coincidences were due to the animal's heightened awareness. Over the years, as I have loosened my grip on my left-brained, scientific training and opened my mind to the possibilities, I am convinced that some pets have abilities that cannot be explained by our current, scientific understanding of animal biology.

We animal lovers are well aware of our pets' ability to sense our moods and comfort us when we are feeling down. There are also cases where pets have been affected by distant deaths and accidents of family members. We have all seen news accounts of pets having warned owners of impending disasters. There are even times when pets have alerted their epileptic owners of an imminent seizure.

From the Cayce readings we learn that psychic ability is a quality of the soul and all people have at least a latent extrasensory capacity.

> Psychic forces, psychic development, are so often misunderstood. Psychic should be applied rather to the soul mind or soul body, than merely to—as is the more often deduced—the *mental* activities of an entity, a soul, a body.
>
> 255-12

Cayce never mentioned the psychic nature of animals but he did make this reference to intuition and animals.

> . . . a concept as would be termed an intuitive force, or through that known as animal telepathic force.   4129-1

A recent book by the scientist Rupert Sheldrake presents credible evidence that pets do have the above-mentioned extrasensory powers. The book is entitled, *Dogs That Know When Their Owners Are Coming Home*. In this book, Sheldrake documents hundreds of cases where animals anticipate the arrival of their owners. He further demonstrates that the animals' predictions cannot be explained by any of the physical senses.

Sheldrake hypothesizes that there is an invisible field, similar to a gravitational field, called a morphic field. This field surrounds and links members of a social group. Theoretically, animals are able to determine situations and events in a way that goes beyond their normal senses by tapping into this field of information. Sheldrake shows how the conjecture of morphic fields explains many other psychic abilities of animals.

Do morphic fields really exist? Are these incredible abilities of animals proof that they have souls? Let's investigate the Cayce readings for their perspective of the animal soul issue.

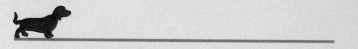

Pet Reincarnation

As seen in the reading about the little dog Mona, which opened this chapter, the Cayce material embraces the concept of reincarnation. We are told that every soul was created by God before time began. We are all sparks of the Eternal Flame. This timeless part of ourselves cycles through the material world, from lifetime to lifetime, to express God's love in this dimension.

Each new lifetime offers us the opportunity to learn from our previous mistakes and build on our triumphs in a continuous process of karma. The cycle proceeds until we reach our final destiny, which is to come to know ourselves to be ourselves and yet one with God.

It is clear in the Cayce readings that, although there is reincarnation of human souls, there is no transmigration. The concept of transmigration, which is held by some Eastern religions, proposes that human souls can come back in animal form. On the contrary, the Cayce material puts forth that mankind is a specialized life form and does not directly commingle with animal life.

In the opening reading for this chapter, 280-1 about Mona, Cayce clearly indicated that she incarnated previously with her owner's husband [280]. She was apparently a lion in the arena of Christian martyrdom fame. Now, there were people who knew Mona who assumed that this reference was an example of the humor that sometimes came through in the readings. Apparently the petite canine fancied herself a lion, with her golden mane and fierce, yapping bark that lifted her off the ground with ferocity.

However, Cayce confirms the previous incarnation of Mona in readings for the dog's owner [286],

> (Q) Where and how have I been formerly associated with
> the following:
> . . . My little dog, Mona?
> (A) In the same experience.
> (Q) In the Roman?
> (A) The Roman.
> (Q) Was she a dog then?
> (A) A lion!   268-3

and the owner's niece [405].

> (Q) In what previous lives have I been associated with the
> following:
> . . . Aunt [268]'s little dog Mona.
> (A) Rome.   405-1

Later in the above exchange we see that the consciousness of animals does cross species boundaries, within the animal kingdom. This point is emphasized by the following question about Mona.

> (Q) Will Mona always be a dog?

(A) That depends upon the environ and the surroundings.
No.   405-1

There was a second pet inquiry that further confirms the Cayce view on animal reincarnation. The following reading segment is for a sixteen-year-old girl asking about her lifetime in ancient Egypt.

(Q) Was the soul-consciousness of Peggy [dog], present in this room, in any of my animals then?
(A) Yes.
(Q) Which one?
(A) In the animals in the home or in the house.   276-6

Again, our exploration has left us with more questions. Why do pets reincarnate? Is it part of their spiritual development? Do they have karmic issues to work out? Have we finally nailed down this soul matter?

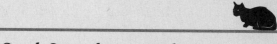

Soul Searching with Cayce

In order to understand the nonphysical anatomy of our pets, we must first have such an appreciation of our own deeper structure. According to Cayce, humans are composed of physical, mental, and spiritual levels. The soul of man partakes both of the mental and spiritual levels. The Cayce readings describe the soul as consisting of Spirit, mind, and will.

Spirit is the life. It is the one and only energy in the universe—the one life force that animates all of creation. We share this aspect with our animal companions as seen in the following exchange.

(Q) Have the lower forms of creation, such as animals, should, or [do they have] any life in the spirit plane?
(A) All have the spirit force.   900-24

Mind is the builder. It gives the vibrational pattern to the life force causing it to manifest physically in various forms. Thus the physical body is the result of the mind's interaction with the Spirit. We also share this feature with our animal friends.

> (Q) Definition of the word *mind*.
> (A) That which is the active force in an animate object; that is the spark, or image of the Maker ...We have the manifestation of this within the lowest order of animal creation.
>
> 3744-2

The mind itself can be understood best if it is viewed as existing on three levels. It has conscious, subconscious, and superconscious aspects. The conscious mind relates to waking, physical consciousness. The subconscious mind is the storehouse of all memories, of both present and past incarnations. The superconscious mind is that part of our consciousness that is still in touch with the infinite Oneness.

Will is our ability to choose how we will work with the mind as we create our physical reality. Let us focus on the will, because Cayce states that our free will is what distinguishes humankind from the animal kingdom.

> ...the will is that factor which makes man different from the rest of the animal kingdom ...   909-1

Because humankind has the ability to choose, this free will creates the opportunity to fulfill our mission in life.

> ...free will—that which is the universal gift to the souls of the children of men; that each entity may know itself to be itself and yet one with the universal cause.   2620-2

Our ability to choose also affords us the capability to go against the Will of God.

Man alone is given that birthright of free will. He alone may
defy his God.   5757-1

In fact the Cayce readings indicate that it is through our choices that
we have distanced ourselves from our creator, choosing to explore our
individualities.

But, what of our companion animals? What are the implications of
being spiritual beings without free will?

Without free-will we become as automatons, or as nature
in its beauty—but ever *just that* expression; while the soul
of man may grow to be equal with, one with, the Creative
Forces.   1435-1

According to the strict Cayce definition of the word soul—consisting
of Spirit, mind, and *will*—animals do not have souls. But, don't let this
statement upset you. It doesn't make the existence of our beloved friends
any less meaningful.

Because mankind has been given the ability to reject the Will of God,
we must use our free will to find our way back to that Oneness. Animals, on the other hand, have not been given free will, so could it be
that they have never left the presence of the Creator? Our will defines
our purpose and our destiny. Animals are obviously on a different mission than we are. Exactly what that mission is, was never touched upon
in the readings. Whatever their purpose, you can bet it is no less
important than our own assignment.

All those forces in nature are fulfilling rather those purposes to which their Maker, their Creator, has called them
into being.   1391-1

Animal Development and Destiny

Even though Copernicus has proven otherwise hundreds of years ago, we humans still feel, both individually and as a group, that we are the center of the universe. We tend to view our universe in our egotistical, anthropocentric way. Other aspects of creation only matter with respect to how they affect us. Our point of view is the right and logical perspective. Our way is the only way. Even our innocently asked question of whether or not animals have souls (just like we have), reveals our human chauvinism.

Well, guess what? Animals as a group and your pet as an individual have a special role to play in the overall scheme of the universe. The creatures of the earth have meaning with or without us. They are developing spiritually and evolving toward their sacred destiny with the rest of creation.

> ... there you have the mineral kingdom, the plant kingdom, the animal kingdom, each developing towards its own source, yet all belonging and becoming one in that force as it develops itself to become one with the Creative Energy, and one with the God.   900-340

Although the Cayce readings indicate that animals lack free will, I have to admit that I have a hard time swallowing the idea myself. My personal experience tells me that there are many strong-willed individuals in the animal kingdom. If our pets lack free will, then by what force do they act? In other words, if they do not choose their actions, then who does?

The readings lead us to believe that animals act strictly out of instinct.

> ... with the desires that are as the instinct in animal for

> the preservation of life, for the development of species,
> and for food. These three are those forces that are instinct
> in the animal and in man.   262-63

So, both human beings and animal beings have the three aspects of instinct—self-preservation, reproduction, and sustenance—in common. Man, however, has the ability to temper his raw instinct through the use of his will. Since animals lack free will, they apparently are ruled strictly by instinct.

Yet, my experience with animals convinces me that these creatures, especially house pets, operate out of more than instinct. If animals were driven only by inborn, genetically programmed reactions, then all individuals would react similarly to the same situation. There are many times that our companion animals' actions defy the three aspects of instinct. Our pets engage in many activities that seem to have nothing to do with food, reproduction, and self-preservation. For instance, why do pets enjoy playing? Also, accounts abound of animals who risk their own lives to save their masters.

If pets do not act from their own free will, perhaps they are influenced by the Will of God. We have seen that their lack of free will precludes them from leaving the presence of God. However, given the brutal and destructive behavior of some animals, this Divine inspiration does not always seem to be in place.

The Cayce readings mention a group consciousness or mind of animals. This explains the coordinated activity displayed by ants and bees and even pack hunters such as wolves. The problem with this concept is that it does not adequately address my experiences with companion animals. It is difficult for me to believe that my dog Louie nuzzles me encouragingly when I am feeling down because of some dog group mind.

Perhaps our pets are influenced by our wills. There may be a kind of group mind within family units, similar to Sheldrake's morphic field concept. Or, maybe our animal companions have evolved since the first half of the twentieth century when Cayce was giving these readings. The spiritual development of our animal friends could be part of the earth changes that Cayce predicted would take place during the current period in history. Possibly, as we have included animals as members of our families, we have influenced their development through the use of *our* minds. It is often stated in the Cayce readings that, "Mind is the builder."

Researchers at the Institute of HeartMath in Boulder Creek, California, have spent over a decade studying the electromagnetic energy generated by the emotions and the heart. By measuring the heart rhythms, they have established that there is an exchange of emotional energy between people. In an informal study, they have further demonstrated such an exchange between a boy and his dog. The pet's heart rhythms changed to match those of his young caregiver when the boy interacted with her, then resumed their original pattern when the boy left the room.

I have noticed through the years in my veterinary practice that pets often reflect the conditions of their owners on many levels. Aggressive people tend to have aggressive pets. Pets are often adversely affected by the stresses their caregivers are going through, even when those conditions do not directly impact the animal. I even see the same medical conditions shared by pet and owner alike. (I sometimes joke that the affliction must run in the family.)

Missy was a wonderful, white Bichon Frisé with gleaming eyes and a cute button nose. She seemed to smile at me every time Mr. and Mrs. Blume brought her in. One day, her mother brought Missy in because she had been vomiting. The poor little thing had lost the spring in her step and her eyes were dull. Her mom did not look well either. Missy groaned as I felt her abdomen. Blood tests revealed that Missy had liver problems. When I told Mrs. Blume the news, she was flabbergasted. "That is so strange," she said, "I was just diagnosed with a liver condition, too." (There was no medical reason for the conditions of these two individuals to be connected.)

I sent Missy home with some medication but lost track of her for a few months. Then one sunny spring day, there were Mrs. Blume and Missy in my exam room. They were both smiling and as bright as ever. The examination showed that Missy was once again in perfect health. I couldn't help but ask Mrs. Blume what had brought about this remarkable change in the two of them. "I got a divorce" was the reply.

You may have expected that I would answer all the questions raised about the nature of our animal friends. Please remember that I will never capture the essence of God's creatures on these pages. As human beings, we each see things from an individual perspective. By our very nature we are biased. As soon as we "know" something, we automatically limit our view. We each have a piece of the puzzle. When we come together, the "big picture" becomes clear. Our animal friends also provide pieces to the puzzle. My goal with this book is to help you "unknow" things so that you may be open to the possibilities afforded by relating to your animal friends. So let us begin the quest to establish a pet connection.

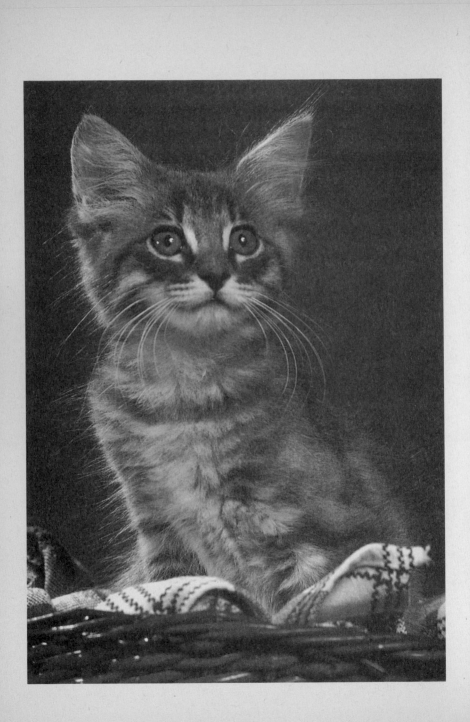

CHAPTER

2

CHOOSING A COMPATIBLE PET

Individuals do not meet by chance. They *are* necessary in the experiences of others, though they may not always use their opportunities in a spiritual way or manner.   2751-1

O ur relationships begin with encountering one another. We are told above, "Individuals do not meet by chance." I believe that this statement applies equally to our animal encounters as it does to our human associations. We attract certain pets into our lives to learn from our relationship with them.

The fact that there are no accidental meetings, however, does not mean that our relationships are predetermined. We have the ability, through the use of our wills, to choose how we will handle the oppor–

tunities presented to us by our animal companions. If we consciously enter the pet selection and relationship process, holding a loving intention, we spiritualize our bonds.

There are many ways to go about choosing a pet. Some people go to a pet store and passionately fall for the cute, cuddly ball of fur that the sales person plops into their hands. Others meticulously research various breeds and breeders to arrive almost mathematically at their selection. Still others take in the stray that wanders up to their doorstep. Certainly, emotions, intellect, and even synchronicity play a role in any conscious decision.

The Edgar Cayce readings add an additional component. They give us several ways of tapping into our intuition for spiritual guidance. These intuition techniques augment our emotions, intellect, and "random" acts of nature to provide a truly holistic animal selection process. They offer a window into the spiritual level of existence that enables us to have a higher view of our lives. Incorporating one or all of these methods into your decision–making will improve your chances of choosing a well–suited pet.

When considering the idea of taking in a pet, it is wise to think things through intellectually before letting emotions and intuition be your guide. All puppies and kitties start out as cute, little bundles of furry fun—then they grow up. Start by narrowing your search down to the right type of pet for your situation and lifestyle. Otherwise a full–time businessperson who works a lot of overtime may end up with a ninety-pound, hyperactive Labrador retriever in a one–bedroom apartment nestled in the middle of a big city. This is obviously not an ideal situation.

They say it takes two to tango, but as the human half of the human–animal equation, *we* are left with the decision as to whether or not to enter into and support a relationship. Certainly, some of our pet connections begin more purposefully than others. Whether you are actively looking for a pet or are just open to the possibility of a pet connection, this chapter will help you in your quest.

We will begin with the practical, intellectual factors that need to be addressed. Later we will explore extrasensory guidance.

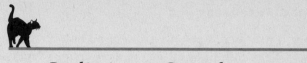

Preliminary Considerations

Before running out to your local pet store, explore the following issues.

Why Do You Want a Pet?

There are many reasons for choosing to start a pet connection. Some people want the protection of a watchdog while others are looking for the affection of a lap cat. Still other folks are trying to replace a lost pet or fill the void left by a broken relationship. Everyone in the household may have a different idea as to the purpose of the pet.

Once a man brought in his eight-week-old beagle for its first exam and vaccines. I asked him about the pup and he said, "Yeah, this is going to be my huntin' dog." Four weeks later his young wife brought the dog in for its next set of shots. I could tell by the way she cuddled and pampered the pooch that it would not be spending its life running through the woods after rabbits.

An individual is likely to have a combination of reasons for keeping a pet. For most of us, the primary motivation for choosing to share our lives with an animal is for the companionship. There is something uncomfortable about coming home to an empty house. A pet adds warmth and life to the cold, barren abode.

Why do you want a pet? Take out a pen and paper right now and write down the reasons—all the reasons. Be sure to involve everyone concerned in the selection process. Get a clear idea of your motivation. Your answers to this question will help to guide you in finding the right companion.

Lifestyle and Resources

Although you may find a pet "free to a good home," keeping a pet takes resources. Selecting the right companion animal depends upon the careful consideration of what you have to offer. Caring for an animal requires time, space, and money. A pet may also cause a change in your lifestyle. Let's look at these factors individually.

Time

The first factor to consider is time. It takes time to properly care for an animal. They are living, breathing, sentient beings. All pets need attention. They thrive on touch and human contact.

This fact is demonstrated by the botched research results for an experiment at Ohio State University. Several groups of rabbits were chosen for research on cholesterol. In preparation for the study, they were all fed a diet high in cholesterol. All the rabbits soon showed high blood cholesterol levels as expected, except one group. This particular group maintained normal blood cholesterol levels even though they were fed the same diet and housed in the same manor as the other bunnies.

As the puzzled researchers sought to explain this anomaly, they discovered that the caregiver for this particular group loved the animals he cared for. Instead of just cleaning the cages and throwing the food in, he would take each rabbit out and pet it. This care and concern was the key factor in why the rabbits stayed healthy.

Having established that all pets need your time and attention, there are some pets that require more than others. Of all the pets out there, dogs require the most time. Canines are pack animals and need lots of social interaction. They need to be taken out for elimination, exercise, and play. Dogs, especially those with long hair coats, require grooming.

Cats require less time and are better suited for people with busy lifestyles. (By the way, for those who do not consider themselves "cat people" I just want to say that I have met many cat lovers who had previously thought that they were not "cat people." It turns out that they had just never lived with a cat before, so they had not developed to their full feline potential.)

It takes time to train young animals. Puppies do not know instinctively that they are supposed to do their business outside. A young dog needs to be taken out every hour to learn what is expected. If the animal is left home alone all day while the owner is at work, it will have no choice but to mess in the house. These early experiences affect the animal's behavior for life.

Litter box training cats is usually not as time consuming. They naturally like to urinate and defecate in dirt or sand. However, cats are more likely to get into and onto things they are not allowed. Vigilant training is needed to stop such behavior. Cats also need to be trained to use the scratching post. This can be a time consuming and frustrating proposition, as some cats prefer the sofa to the scratching post.

It also takes a certain amount of time to clean up after any pet. All dogs and cats shed, but longhaired individuals tend to be "hair factories" and you may find yourself running the vacuum more often. Cats need to have their litter boxes kept clean and even though dogs do their business outside, you'll need to clean up their messy land mines from the yard.

Are you willing to commit the time needed to care for a pet? If not, get a stuffed animal.

Space

When choosing a pet, you need to consider the space requirements. Common sense dictates that the larger the pet, the more space is required. A small apartment works well for a cat or small breed dog, but not for a large dog. Cats are better off when kept indoors, but dogs need time outdoors. For the canines you either need a large, fenced-in yard or plenty of time to take them for leash walks several times a day.

For people who live in rented property, it is important to keep in mind that not all landlords allow pets. Although this may not be a factor in your current situation, if you need to move for some reason, owning a pet can limit your choices. It breaks my heart to see the number of animals left at shelters every year due to a move by the owner.

Money

It costs money to own a pet. Food and other care items add up, and then there are medical bills. Most of us are not used to paying medical bills because we have insurance. Medical costs for animals are much lower than those for humans but they still can be significant.

A recent survey of pet owners done by the American Veterinary Medical Association found that in the first year of a puppy or kitten's life the average pet owner will spend $900 on a kitten and $1500 on a puppy. This includes the cost of food and medical care but not the actual purchase price.

Are you willing to put your money where your pet is?

Lifestyle

Caring for an animal companion is a life–long commitment. We've just discussed some of the challenges involved in pet ownership. Now let us look at issues that concern your personal convenience.

Remember that if you are planning to add an additional pet to your household, you need to consider how your plans will affect the lifestyles of other animals you are already caring for. Some pets enjoy being an "only child" and although most will eventually warm up to the new family member, some never do. The situation with cats is especially tricky. In general, cats are less pack oriented and more territorial than dogs are. The more cats you get in the same house, the more likely are such behavior problems as urinating out of the box and destructive scratching. Of course, any animal that has not been socialized with other pets at a young age is likely to have difficulties adjusting to having another pet in the house.

Pet owners who are on the go need to have a plan for the care of their pets while they are gone. For many people the answer is kennel-ing. More and more kennels are catering to the pampered pet and offer accommodations that are akin to vacation suites with activities for the animals. There are even puppy daycare centers available for short–term animal care. These are viable choices for many pet owners but carry the risk of spread of disease. Also, no matter how posh the living condi-tions, it's never the same as the animal's home, and some pets prefer their familiar surroundings.

Another option for pet care is to keep the animal home and rely on family or neighbors to watch them. I have clients who swap services with their neighbors, each caring for the others pets as needed. There are also professional pet sitters who come to the home and walk and care for pets. All of these options are subject to availability and are not always reliable.

The bottom line is that caring for an animal requires planning for the care of the pet in the owner's absence. Of course, the care may involve taking the pet with you. This opens a whole new area of possibilities and problems. Many people enjoy their vacations with their pets. How-ever, consideration must be taken as to accommodations that will allow pets. Not all hotels accept pets. You also need to plan for the care of the pet while the family is enjoying a restricted activity. For example, what do you do with Fido when the family spends the day at the museum?

Besides the challenges of travel, it must be remembered that animals do not stay young and healthy forever. As animals age, they sometimes develop debilitating diseases and require much more attention. Are you willing to give an animal what it needs even when it becomes extremely inconvenient?

A further consideration is that the average dog or cat may live to be twelve to fifteen years of age or even older. When you choose a puppy or kitten you are committing yourself to at least a decade of care. Where do you see yourself fifteen years from now? How will an old pet fit into your lifestyle then?

What Kind of Pet?

So, in spite of the commitment, you are determined to initiate a pet connection. Then, now it is time to begin narrowing down your choices. Before zeroing in on a specific animal, let's begin by exploring all of our options by examining the general categories of pets.

Reptiles, Pocket Pets, Birds, Fish

Although I focus mostly on dogs and cats as companions in this book, I would like to mention the pros and cons of keeping smaller animals as pets. These smaller pets are an alternative for people who are allergic to dogs and cats. They have the advantage of providing company without taking up much room. Most can be kept in a small cage or aquarium, yet many people are surprised by how much personality and affection such animals exhibit. However, in spite of their small size, the husbandry of these creatures often requires as much time as caring for a dog or cat. Each one of these pets has unique health requirements that need to be met.

It is essential that the animal lover do research before and not after acquiring any pet. It is also important to realize that veterinary care for birds and exotic pets has gotten quite specialized in the last few decades. Many veterinarians who have not kept up with the recent advances refuse to treat these more unusual pets all together. Be sure to locate a good avian/exotic veterinarian nearby before you run into pet health problems.

Some people are really drawn to reptiles. I have met people who have formed strong relationships with these scaly creatures. However, I do not recommend keeping snakes or lizards unless you really know what you are doing. Reptiles have very specific requirements for housing, lighting, and food. It is difficult for most people to mimic Mother Nature in the way that these animals need. The majority of health conditions that I see in captive reptiles are brought on by the ignorance of the creature's caregiver.

There are numerous small mammals, such as rabbits, guinea pigs, ferrets, chinchillas, hedgehogs, gerbils, hamsters, mice, and rats that can be ideal pets for certain people. Of the above-mentioned animals, I find that guinea pigs especially are cute and cuddly and somewhat hardy pets. They don't take up much room and do not require a lot of care. Rabbits, too, can fill the bill. I've met some that were litter trained and were left to run freely around the house. A guinea pig or rabbit can make the perfect companion for a busy apartment dweller.

Birds are unique creatures and can brighten any home with their airy energy. Small birds like budgies, canaries, finches, and cockatiels are quite affordable and require little space. Although the smaller birds are not known for talking, they still can make a perfect companion for the right person. The large parrots on the other hand can be quite expensive and require more care. All birds tend to be messy with their seeds and food. Hand-raised birds are generally tamer and easier to handle than those captured from the wild.

For those animal lovers with little time or space, consider the virtues of keeping tropical fish. It is true that these scaly aquatic dwellers are not as cuddly as more traditional pets, yet studies have shown that just watching them glide through the water can lower a person's blood pressure. After the initial setup costs, the expense associated with aquarium care is quite affordable for anyone. Once established, an aquarium is easy to care for and fish do not require grooming or walking and they never bring fleas into the house. Also, tropical fish are a great startup pet for kids, teaching them the basics of animal care without overwhelming them with responsibility.

Dogs

Dogs are considered by many to be "man's best friend." Perhaps this is because our relationship with dogs goes way back. The conventional view is that man began to domesticate wolves 10,000 to 20,000 years ago. However, recent DNA evidence suggests that the process may have begun as early as 100,000 years ago. Human evolution is deeply intertwined with that of our canine friends.

Dogs have a social structure that we can easily relate to. They quickly adopt a family as their pack. Their social interaction within the family-pack elicits a strong attachment from their human companions.

Our canine friends seem to want nothing more than to please us. Most are easily trained when the right techniques are applied. Dogs love to play and interact with family members. Intensive breeding has created breeds of every shape and size. There are few people who cannot find some dog to brighten their days.

Cats

Cats are unique individuals. They began their symbiotic relationship with man about 5,000 years ago in Egypt. The common denominator for this liaison was grain. Early human city dwellers stored grain which attracted rodents. People found cats useful as pest control agents. The felines tolerated us because our habit of hoarding food attracted their favorite cat chow.

For cats, the association with humans remains one of mutual respect. Those who are fortunate enough to have been taken in by a stray cat know what I'm talking about. Cats have the reputation of being nonsocial creatures, but this is not usually the case. They do tend to be more independent than dogs, yet in general they love to interact with other animals, as well as the people in the household.

It is important to realize that the statements made about the characteristics of dogs and cats are generalizations. Just like our children, each individual animal is self determined and may possess traits that are not common to the species as a whole. For instance, there are particular dogs that are standoffish and independent, and some cats that have more social, dog-like personalities.

This same consideration is true of breeds of dogs and cats as well. You may read that Labrador Retrievers are friendly and that Rottweilers are aggressive. Although these statements are true for the most part, I have met a few aggressive Labs and many friendly Rottweilers. Certain breeds of cats have their notorious characteristics as well and yet individuals have their own personalities. Keep this in mind as we explore factors involved in choosing the ideal dog or cat.

Selecting the Ideal Dog or Cat

When choosing a companion, one of the first considerations is whether to get a young animal or an adult. There are pros and cons to caring for each age group so weigh the possibilities carefully. You also need to consider what type of pet suits you best—the perfect purebred or the mighty mutt. Either kind can make a great pet so the choice is yours.

Puppies/Kittens

Puppies and kittens are cute and cuddly but the real advantage to starting off with a young companion is that you have control over the pet's socialization and bonding during the critical, first few months of age. The way a dog or cat is treated and what they are exposed to during the first three to four months of age determine how they will behave for the rest of their lives. All of the training in the world cannot undo the damage done to a puppy or kitten by improper socialization.

The importance of these first few months also explains the disadvantage of caring for a puppy. It takes a lot of time and energy to properly train and socialize a young dog. A puppy needs to be trained to obey and to poop and pee outside. Puppies need to be taken out every thirty to sixty minutes for the first few months to be house trained. It is true that you can teach them to go on newspapers, but then you have to totally retrain them to go outside when they get older. A puppy is not a good pet for a household where no one is home all day during this critical training period.

Kittens are a little easier than puppies. Most kittens take to the litter box almost by instinct, although no good behavior should be taken for granted. It is not as important for cats to learn certain commands as it is for dogs. One area of training that is important for kittens is the use of the scratching post. Left on its own, a kitten may choose any surface to scratch. It is up to the owner to guide the kitten to a scratching post and not the furniture.

Even with the best of intentions, genetics, and training techniques, you never quite know for sure just how a puppy or kitten is going to turn out. Will this cute little Golden Retriever puppy grow to be fifty pounds or one hundred and twenty pounds? Will this cuddly Persian turn into a lap cat or a wild cat. Will that spunky little creature settle down or be hyperactive for life? Each animal comes into this earth with its own agenda. This is where the spiritual guidance techniques described later in the chapter can help to intuitively match your ideals with those of your animal companion.

Another consideration about choosing a puppy or kitten is that they are more fragile than an adult pet. A juvenile animal may not be the ideal pet for a family with small children, who can easily hurt a puppy or kitten with inappropriate treatment. At the other end of the spectrum, puppies and kittens tend to be clingy and often get under the feet of the caregiver. This propensity makes them ill-suited for an elderly owner because of the risk of the senior being tripped and injured by the youngster.

It takes a lot of energy to keep up with a growing animal. They are so active and curious, and they tend to get into everything. Just like children, puppies and kittens want to put everything they see in their mouths. Electrical cords, poisonous plants, even your favorite pair of shoes—nothing is too dangerous or too sacred to bite, chew, and possibly swallow. Living with a young animal is not for those who are impatient.

Adult Dogs/Cats

Adult dogs and cats are not as cute as their younger counterparts, but they are sturdier. Also, much of the training hassle can be avoided by adopting a full-grown dog or cat—that is assuming the animal has been well trained and socialized by the previous owner. This is not an assumption you want to take for granted.

Adopting an adult dog or cat has the advantage of knowing exactly what you will end up with. What you see is what you get. The key is that you need to be sure of what you are looking at. Sure, you can make out what he looks like and how he behaves under the conditions in which you are viewing him. One important question is, "How will this beautiful animal behave in your home environment?" Does the dog walk well on a leash? Will he be territorial and bite strangers, including your children's playmates? Will he be defensive of his food and attack anyone who comes near him while he is eating? Is the cat in a habit of clawing the furniture and stealing food off the table?

These questions can only be answered by seeing the animal's response to these particular situations. You need to get as much information as you can from the current caretaker of the pet. I also advise that you not commit to the dog or cat until you have personally tested his temperament in your home environment. Take the pet on a trial basis and put him through his paces.

Pedigrees

The advantage of selecting a purebred animal is that each breed has certain general characteristics that you can usually count on. Breed-related personality traits are more dependable in dogs than cats. Golden Retrievers tend to be gentle and good with kids while Pit Bulls tend to be aggressive. Of course, there are exceptions to these tendencies. Pedigrees of both dogs and cats do give the certainty of appearance. Persian cats have long hair coats and pug noses, Siamese cats have short fur and long noses, and if you buy a Dalmatian puppy you can bet that when it grows up it will have spots.

Ninety percent of American cat owners have mixed breed animals. It appears that most cat fanciers value *purr*sonality over pedigree. Mixed breed cats come in a collection of colors, a plethora of patterns, and a selection of hair styles. There are at least two cats to please every cat-lover's eyes. Of course, the fact that, when left to their own devices, wild cats are very prolific breeders adds to their abundance. Since supply outstrips demand, mixed breed cats can usually be found "free to a good home," which adds to their popularity. Besides, who can resist the cute, little face and longing cries of an abandoned kitten?

On the other hand, many people have a particular breed of dog in mind as they seek a new pet. Unfortunately, our fetish for a certain type of dog is too often influenced by what we see on TV or in movies. These animal movie stars are portrayed in home settings, giving the viewer the impression that this is how a typical individual of that breed is likely to behave at home. In reality, the most trainable dog is selected and tirelessly trained by a professional. Then we have to remember that what we see as a typical afternoon on the screen is actually a series of scenes that has been filmed over days or weeks, and any footage of less-than-ideal animal behavior ends up on the cutting room floor.

A case in point is that Jack Russell Terriers have gained in popularity in recent years. It is no secret that the reason for this breed's sudden attractiveness is because of Eddie on the hit TV show *Frazier*. In this comedy series, Eddie is a cute, witty, little, well-mannered dog with lots of personality. Who could resist such an animal companion? The truth is that Jack Russells are notoriously strong-willed, aggressive, hyperactive, little powerhouses that can be difficult to train. People are often disappointed with the results when they choose a pet based on what they see on TV.

Sometimes people choose a particular breed because of past personal experience with a pet of that breed. This is a step up from picking a movie star dog, but once again it is essential to appreciate that each individual has her own personality. Just because your childhood Cocker Spaniel was a wonderful pet does not mean that the one in the pet store window will grow up to behave the same way.

If you have to have a purebred animal, the best starting point for choosing a breed is to get some books and do some research. There are many books available that help differentiate the distinguishing characteristics of the many types of dogs and cats. One such book for dogs is, *The Right Dog for You* by Daniel F. Tortora, Ph.D. It even grades each breed on such things as obedience, sociability, and emotional stability.

Once a breed is selected, the question often arises as to where to go for the dog or cat. I think your best bet is to find a local, reputable breeder. The internet is a great resource for information on breeders. You should also talk to people you see with the breed in question. Dog and cat magazines can help, too. Local kennel clubs and cat fanciers clubs may be of assistance in locating a breeder as well. Be sure to see the premises and the parents of the puppies or kittens, as well as contacting owners of pets from previous litters.

Pet stores are another source of purebred dogs and cats. Unfortunately, pet store dogs are often the product of "puppy mills" where inbreeding and poor conditions result in unhealthy pets. This seems to be less of a problem with the kitties. However, even if the pets come from a good breeder, you can bet that only the reject animals are sold to the pet store. In fact, if you read the information from the pet store carefully, you will often find the statement that the animals are "pet quality." When purchasing a dog or cat from a pet store, be sure to find out where he came from and who the breeder was. Ask to see the pedigrees of both parents and also ask for references from satisfied customers. If this information is not available, find a reputable pet store.

Besides the health issues involved with the breeding situation of many pet store puppies and kitties, most pet store managers, in their zeal to sell healthy animals, overvaccinate and overmedicate the pets creating the opposite condition. The conventional view is that the more vaccines a pet receives, the healthier it is likely to be. As we will see in chapter 5, this is not the case.

An additional resource for purebred dogs—usually adults—is a local rescue group. Many popular breeds have a rescue group that tries to find homes for unwanted pets of that particular type. These volunteers are moved by their love for the breed and do their best to match the right dog with the right owner. They want the relationship to work out so they get to know the animals and warn the prospective owner of any incompatible traits of the pet. To locate such a group, contact you local pet shelter or check with your veterinarian.

A question that arises when dealing with purebred animals is what to do with the registration papers. Registering your pet as a purebred is only important if you plan to use it for breeding. I strongly recommend against breeding unless you really know what you are doing. Many breeds have trouble delivering their young and need C-sections. This emergency surgery can easily cost $1,000.00 and you may be risking the life of your pet. Any good breeder will tell you that there are many other hidden costs associated with the business. Most breeders are in it not for the money but out of love for the breed.

The Underdog

There is a concept in biology known as hybrid vigor. A hybrid animal is the offspring of adults of different types—with very different genetic material. An example of a hybrid would be any mixed-breed dog or cat. The idea of hybrid vigor is that such an animal would be more likely to thrive than a purebred pet.

Here's how it works. Many times, the genes for undesirable, genetic defects lie dormant or recessive. Closely related individuals have more genes (genetic material) in common. They are more likely to be carrying the same defective genes and their mating has a higher likelihood of producing offspring with genetic flaws.

Mankind has developed purebred animals by interbreeding closely related individuals that have desired characteristics (such as the spots on Dalmatians). Because of this inbreeding, by their very natures purebred animals are more likely to be plagued by genetic defects. These flaws can range from hardly noticeable, such as crooked teeth, to fatal, such as heart defects.

In fact, the "art" of breeding has gotten to the point today that some breeders are obsessed by the conformation of their breeding stock while ignoring their personalities. It doesn't matter if the animal is hyperactive or aggressive, as long as they look acceptable to the judge in the show ring. The more frequently hyperactive or aggressive pets are used for breeding, the more common those traits become in the population of purebred animals.

Now certainly not all breeders are bad and not all purebred pets are defective. I also do not mean to imply that all mixed breeds have strong constitutions. But the fact is that the common mutt is likely to live a longer, healthier life. Let's hear it for the underdog! Some of the best pets can be saved from certain death and obtained rather inexpensively from a local pet shelter.

There are a couple of precautions about adopting a shelter pet. First of all, you never know the background of the animal. Was it abused? Was it well nourished? For young animals these are important questions because the social behavior of dogs and cats depends on how they were treated as youngsters. Major aberrations in the socialization of a youngster may affect it for life no matter what you do to correct the problems. Severe, early malnutrition can cause physical problems for the entire life of a pet. This is a less common situation but needs to be considered when choosing any pet.

For those considering adopting an older pet from a shelter, a key question is, "Why was the pet discarded?" Many pets are brought to a shelter because of behavioral difficulties. Unfortunately, people dropping off a pet for such a reason are reluctant to confess this to the shelter personnel, so they are likely to make up some other excuse. The good news is that many "behavioral" problems are due to the pet owner and not the pet.

Another concern when adopting a pet from a shelter is the health of the pet. Many pets at the shelter have not been raised in favorable conditions. They are almost never vaccinated properly, which leaves them wide open to be infected by life–threatening viruses. Many health problems are obvious and can be easily detected. However, some viral infections, such as Parvo in puppies, do not start making the pet sick for seven to ten days after the animal was exposed. A puppy could become infected, be dropped off at the shelter and adopted by an unsuspecting Good Samaritan, then get sick the next day. I don't know of a way around this hazard.

The most common mistake people make when adopting a pet is that they feel sorry for a sickly animal. As pitiful as the sickly, runt of the litter may look, I wouldn't recommend it for a pet unless you have unlimited financial and emotional resources. There is nothing more heartbreaking that losing a youngster after pouring all your love and attention into her.

As harsh as it may seem, you need to realize the cold reality of the animal shelter. Many of the animals you see at the shelter will be put to sleep. In fact, such euthanasia is the biggest cause of death for pets at large. You can't save them all so you may as well focus on a thriving pet. If you select an unhealthy pet it only means that one of the healthy ones you didn't choose will be killed. When rooting for the underdog, don't set your sights too low.

Temperament

Every animal has its own personality and temperament. They each have their own unique style of interacting with others. The disposition of an adult is a result of genetics, its innate spirit, and its early life experiences. The first two factors are set at birth and the third is irreversible by five months of age. No matter what the age, it is imperative to evaluate the animal's temperament before taking it in.

When choosing a pet from a litter, first observe how the youngster behaves among her siblings. Is she domineering, does she hide in the corner of the pen, or is she playing give and take with the rest of the group? If you want an aggressive, outgoing pet choose pet number one. If you want a shy, couch potato that may hide from strangers choose the second. For most people, the third is the best choice. She is most likely to be easily trainable with an even temper.

Next, check out how each animal interacts with other people who are with you. The same considerations as above apply. If the pet is aggressive now, it will likely maintain that temperament throughout life. If she starts out shy, you may never get her to come out of her shell. Once again, the middle of the road animal suits most people the best.

Finally, see how each youngster individually reacts to you alone. Does she come to you without being coaxed? Does she run away or ignore you? When you hold her, does she fight you, play with you, or lie in your hands like a lump? As you hold each pet, close your eyes, take slow, deep breaths, and focus your attention on the creature in your hands. How does she *feel*? Let your intuition be your guide.

Health Check

It is best to start off with a healthy pet. A relationship with a new creature can be challenging enough without starting out behind the eight ball. To be sure of the health status of the animal you need to use close, directed observation.

Objectively look at the pet. What is her level of vitality? Do you see any limping or trouble moving? Does her hair coat look normal? Look at every square inch. Are there any bald spots, sores, fleas, or ticks? Run your fingers against the grain of the fur to check for tiny, black, comma–shaped flea dirt. Where there is flea dirt, there are fleas. It only takes a few of these parasites on a puppy or kitten to drink a life–threatening amount of blood.

Now, start at the front and work your way back. Check the eyes. Are they clear and bright? Is there a discharge or tearing? Is there any dis–charge from the nose or any sneezing? Problems with the eyes and nose can be a sign of respiratory problems. Upper respiratory infections can develop into a nagging, life–long condition in certain cats.

Open the mouth to check the teeth. Also check the roof of the mouth for cleft palate. This birth defect results in an opening between the mouth and nasal passages which can result in the youngster literally inhaling food or drink and developing pneumonia.

Look on the inside and around the outside of each ear. A dark dis–charge is usually a sign of ear mites or other ear infection. Sores around the ears usually indicate that the pet has been scratching the ears due to some type of irritation or infection.

Check the body for any bumps or swellings. In the center of the underside, just behind the rib cage is the umbilicus or belly button. Any swelling at this point is a sign of a hernia. An inguinal hernia appears as a swelling in the groin area where the back leg meets the body. A pot–bellied appearance usually indicates worms.

Finally, check under the tail for any signs of loose stool stuck to the fur. Such a finding indicates diarrhea and possible health concerns. While you're back there, confirm the sex of the pet and for males, be sure that the testicles have descended into the scrotum.

If the pet passes inspection, great! If not, weigh the health conditions against the attributes of the animal. Don't necessarily disqualify a puppy because of ear mites, fleas, or worms. These are usually minor problems that can be easily remedied. A few such parasites are common and are usually more an indication of lack of care by the pet's owner than the weakness of the animal.

All of the above, left–brained criteria for choosing a pet are very important considerations. The human intellect is a powerful tool when it comes to decision making. At the same time, basing any choice strictly on the hard, cold facts usually leads to unpleasant results. This is especially true when the judgment involves a relationship. Our intuition is an equally valuable tool when seeking to draw the perfect pet into our lives.

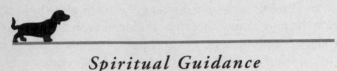

Spiritual Guidance

In order to enter into a pet connection in a holistic manner, we must engage all aspects of our beings. We must honor the physical, mental, and spiritual sides of ourselves and the animal kingdom. Certainly we are influenced by spiritual forces whether we are aware of it or not. However, the more consciously we engage this influence in decision making, the more satisfied we will be with the results of the choice and the more sense any challenges that may arise will make.

> The more and more each is impelled by that which is intuitive, or the relying upon the soul force within, the greater, the farther, the deeper, the broader, the more constructive may be the result.   792-2

The Cayce readings are a great resource for learning how to cultivate spiritual guidance in our lives. In fact, the readings encourage people to develop their own psychic abilities. In this sense, Cayce was using the original definition of the word psychic which literally means "of the soul." So psychic abilities are a result of an established connection with the divine. We all have extrasensory capabilities because we all have this connection.

I am sure you can recall times that you thought of someone and just then that person called on the phone. Or perhaps you have had a gut feeling that turned out to be accurate. The question is how to tap this ability at will. More specifically, how can we use our innate psychic abilities to help with the decision of choosing the right pet? Certainly Cayce had an exceptional ability to enter a state of psychic attunement and tap this spiritual source of information. At the same time, the readings suggest several ways for us to get in touch with the unseen forces. In fact, we all unwittingly enter such a state every night when we fall asleep and dream.

Dreaming Up a Pet

When we sleep, our physical bodies are quiet and our consciousness loses its close association with the material world. Quite naturally we become aware of the deeper levels of mind and spirit through our dreams. It is a strange world of symbols and often bizarre activities. As ordinary and confusing as dreams may seem, they are our most easily accessible way of contacting higher levels of awareness. In order to use our dreams constructively for spiritual guidance, we need to explore the process step by step. Here is one way to work with your dreams.

1. The first step to using dreams for guidance is to realize that whether or not you remember your dreams, research leaves no doubt that we all do dream each night. By monitoring the electrical activity of the brain, scientists have discovered that as people sleep, they cycle in and out of several patterns of brain waves. They have labeled one such pattern REM sleep because of the rapid eye movement that always accompanies it.

Researchers have determined that we dream during REM sleep. Furthermore, subjects who are deprived of the dream phase of sleep soon develop severe psychological problems. These psychotic conditions are easily reversed by once again allowing the subjects to dream. So, as long as you are not psychotic you can be sure that you do dream. At the same time, remembering our dreams can be tricky.

2. The second step for obtaining dream guidance is to work on dream recall. Why is it that some of us have difficulty remembering our dreams? Dreams seem to be made of very fragile material. As you awaken you lie there in bed, reveling in a fantastic dream. Suddenly the alarm goes off, you get ready for work, and in the car you remember that you had a wonderful dream but have no idea what it was about.

We dream at a level of consciousness that is beyond our waking awareness. The Cayce readings and other sources describe layers of the mind—conscious, subconscious, and superconscious. The barriers between these mental levels can be so dense that one part does not know what the others are up to. Our dreams occur at the subconscious and superconscious levels while we function in the world at the conscious level. Once we move fully into our conscious minds, the dream is left behind on the other side.

In order to pull a dream through the barrier between the conscious and subconscious minds we must ease the transition from the dream world to the waking state. When you first wake up, just lie there and allow your mind to rest a moment. Think about what was just happening in your mind. Before engaging the body and getting out of bed, write down any impressions and images that come up. Often, as you begin to write, more of the dream will reveal itself.

Another surefire way to remember dreams and get guidance is to engage your desire. It is as if your mind needs a reason to remember dreams—you never paid any attention to them in the past. To convince your mind that you want to remember your dreams and that you intend to take them seriously you need to have a purpose. Presently, you want to have a dream to help you attract the perfect pet for you.

The process involved is call dream incubation. You simply ask for a dream to assist you. As you drift off to sleep, repeat to yourself the following affirmation, "I will awaken in the morning refreshed and remembering a dream that will help me attract the best pet for me." The affirmation acts as a pre–sleep suggestion that activates your subconscious mind to carry out your wish. I find that when I dream for a purpose, my subconscious mind invariably hands me a memorable story in the morning.

3. Of course, remembering and transcribing a dream is only half the battle. The third step for dream guidance is figuring out what it means. There are entire books written about dream interpretation, and psychologists and seekers alike have spent their entire lives unlocking the mysteries of these nocturnal visions. It is beyond the scope of this book to act as a dream guide, but here are a few pointers from the Cayce readings to get you started.

Begin by exploring the dominant emotion of the dream. How did it make you feel and where does that feeling match a situation in your waking life? Now look at the theme of the dream. Make up a title such as "Someone Travels from One Place to Another," leaving out names and details. Lastly, view the people and images in the dream as symbols. What does the secret code mean to you? Try to run through this process quickly as you are just waking up and still in touch with your deeper self. Your own subconscious mind is the best interpreter of your dreams.

4. The final step to encourage dream guidance is to actually use whatever information you get from your dreams. Even if you cannot figure out the dream's exact meaning, use what you do know. Doodle some of the symbols and put the paper in your pocket or on your desk. If all you get is a color, wear something with that color. Find some way to put into practice what you experienced in the dream. Realize that the full meaning of any message from within may gradually unfold as you wrestle with it. The implication often becomes clear as a significant life situation occurs.

This is just a rudimentary look at how to handle dreams. For a more complete explanation and more techniques I recommend reading *Dream Interpretation (AND MORE) Made Easy* by Kevin J. Todeschi.

Meditation

The Cayce readings tout meditation as a more purposeful way of connecting with the Divine within. For some, the thought of meditation may conjure up the image of an emaciated holy man donning turban and robes and sitting cross-legged, chanting "Om" for hours. Certainly there are many forms of meditation and ways to look at it. Research indicates that meditation relaxes the body, helping to lower blood pressure, reduce insomnia, relieve headaches and chronic pain, and even slow the aging process. Other researchers have found that meditation reduces anxiety, improves test taking, and promotes creativity. There are even studies demonstrating that groups of people meditating in unison can reduce violent crimes in their surrounding area.

So, just what is meditation? Let's see what the Cayce readings have to say.

> Meditation is listening to the Divine within.   1861-19

> [Meditation] is not musing, not daydreaming . . . it is the attuning of the mental body and the physical body to its spiritual source.   281-41

> *Meditation is emptying* of self of all that hinders the creative forces from rising along the natural channels of the physical man to be disseminated through those centers and sources that create the activities of the physical, the mental, the spiritual man; properly done must make one *stronger* mentally, physically . . .   281-13

The Cayce approach to meditation emphasizes the inner process, the tuning in to that Divine presence within. All of the physical and mental benefits are simply the side effects of strengthening this connection.

So, just how do we go about meditating? Once again, space will allow me only a brief description of the process. There are many books written about the Cayce method of meditation. My personal favorite is Mark Thurston's *The Inner Power of Silence*. As that title suggests, the practice of meditation involves quieting the body and mind. Here are steps to follow for a simple meditation.

1. Posture—Sit upright in a straight-backed chair with your back straight to maintain spinal alignment. Have your feet flat on the floor and legs uncrossed. Allow your hands to rest comfortably in your lap. Keep your head in an erect position. You want the body to be at ease but not so relaxed as to fall asleep.

2. Relax—Close your eyes and breathe deeply and slowly. With each inhalation feel peace and relaxation enter your body. With each exhalation feel the tension and worries of the day fade away. Feel the muscles of your body relax. With each breath allow the relaxation to spread and deepen.

3. Prayer—The Cayce material recommends starting with a prayer of protection to guide your consciousness from distractions. One such prayer from the readings is, "As I approach the throne of grace, beauty, and might, I surround myself with the protection found in the thought of the Christ." The Lord's Prayer is also appropriate at this time. These are usually prayed in silence.

4. Affirmation—An affirmation is a phrase that is repeated to evoke a feeling. The feeling we are attempting to foster is one of peace, upliftment, and oneness with whatever concept we have of God or the Divine. A good phrase for our purposes is, "Be still and know God." It is often helpful to link the affirmation to the breath. As you exhale say to yourself, "Be still." Feel the stillness in your body and mind. Imagine your body as a perfectly calm pool, or use whatever imagery helps you get the feeling. With the next exhalation say, "And know God." Feel the presence of the Divine. Imagine light, warmth, and love flooding over and through your body. Bask in the enlightening sensation. As the feeling fades or as distracting thoughts arise, simply repeat the affirmation.

5. End—When you feel the time is right, gently take a few deep breaths and bring your awareness back to your surroundings. Wiggle your fingers and toes. There is no set time allotment for meditation. You can go through the above steps in just a few minutes or you can extend the period to last an hour or more. For most beginners, ten to twenty minutes works well. Before ending the session, take the energy that you just raised and channel it in the form of prayers for others.

This is also a good time to ask for guidance. Simply ask your question and quietly remain open for a response. Realize that the response may come as a word, a picture or a feeling. If you do not get a clear "Yes" or "No" or a tap on the shoulder do not be concerned. You have put the question out there and the answer will come. It may come in the form of synchronistic events or conversations. It may come in days, weeks or years, but it will come.

As you can see, meditation for guidance does not mean meditating on a problem or question. We don't go over and over the question in our minds and try to reason it out. Rather, we attune to the highest source of wisdom, ask our question, and then wait for the answer.

The Cayce readings clearly state that when using meditation for guidance, it is best to do your homework first. Before the meditation go through the intellectual process of making the decision, weighing the pros and cons carefully, and coming up with an answer. Then, after meditation, ask for confirmation of your judgment.

This technique can be used at every decision point in the process of choosing the ideal pet for you. You can ask, "I have decided to get a cat, is this an ideal decision?" Then, after more consideration ask, "I have decided to get a kitten from the humane society, is this ideal?" You can then take this method down to the final decision of which kitten to choose. This can be done in a less formal way while holding the prospective pet. Just close your eyes, relax, feel the presence, and ask.

Prayer and Affirmations

Another way of asking for divine guidance is with prayer. Where as meditation is often thought of as listening to God, prayer is seen as speaking to God. In the West we are much more familiar with prayer than we are with meditation. We have prayers of praise and thanksgiving, intercessory prayers, formal prayers, informal prayers, and ritualistic prayers. Prayers for healing have even been the subject for scientific studies. Time after time in very formal experiments, the power of prayer has proven effective, much to the chagrin of some scientists.

Just how does prayer work? Physical science cannot explain it. Again, let's turn to the Cayce readings for elucidation of the subject.

> ... prayer is the *making* of one's conscious self more in attune with the spiritual forces that may manifest in a material world ... Prayer is the concerted effort of the physical consciousness to become attuned to the consciousness of the Creator, either collectively or individually!   281-13

Just like meditation, prayer involves an attunement, a connection with the Divine.

And, just like meditation, prayer involves a feeling; in this case it is a feeling of expectancy. Jesus stated it clearly:

> "Therefore I tell you, whatever you ask for in prayer, believe that you have received it, and it will be yours."
>
> (Mark 11:24 NIV)

To pray effectively we must hold a feeling that our needs have already been met—a sense of faith. It is the feeling of walking into the unknown blindfolded and moving forward with the confidence that with each step our foot will fall upon solid support. This is the mustard seed–sized faith that can move mountains.

Even if we can't seem to muster enough faith to move a mountain, certainly we can gather enough to move a pet into our lives. How can we do this? Simply by holding in our hearts a feeling that the right pet is already headed our way. The prayer might go something like this, "Heavenly Father–Mother God, creator of all beasts, large and small, thank You for drawing to me the perfect pet for the best of all involved."

It is important to hold an intention that acknowledges the value of others' experiences as well as your own. Your true motives are known to the universe, and selfish prayers may result in difficult lessons. An ideal pet is one who gains as much from the relationship as you and your family do.

From the age of two, Pat's nightly prayers included a petition for a puppy. However, her parents continually refused all requests for a dog, citing the added work and danger of their suburban street to a wandering canine. Over the years she resolved her fate, but her prayers had been heard and laid up in heaven.

When Pat and her husband married and built their new log home on ten wooded acres in the middle of farm country, she excitedly assumed she could now get a puppy. Her husband disagreed, stating that their long work hours would be completely unfair to a dog. Case closed!

Several years into her marriage, Pat began to feel her biological clock ticking furiously. She felt overwhelmed with the need to love and nurture something. Starting a family was out of the question, and one afternoon Pat found herself having a talk with God on her drive home from work. She said, "Lord, if You don't give me someone to nurture and love, I'll just burst!"

A short time later as she was driving home from work, Pat noticed a beautiful caramel-colored Cocker Spaniel running loose on her road. Being that she lived so far out in the country and had so few neighbors, Pat knew most of the family pets in her area. This little dog was a stranger and looked lost.

Concerned for his safety, Pat pulled over and called to him. He ran right up and happily joined her on the front seat. She was delighted and quickly determined that he had no collar or tags. She started home with her newfound friend. It seemed her prayers had finally been answered.

Then qualms of conscience started to pierce her heart. This little guy was clean, well fed, and obviously loved by a family somewhere. Even though no one would ever discover her new "pet" that she so desperately desired, Pat knew she had to do the right thing.

The lady at the police station recognized the dog immediately. As she handed the lost pooch over, Pat assured the woman that if he went unclaimed she would keep him. When Pat called the dispatcher the next morning and learned that her little friend had indeed found his home, she felt good that she had done the right thing, but she longed for a dog of her own all the more.

About a month later, after a weekend outing, Pat rose at 6:00 a.m. Monday morning and started downstairs to make breakfast. As she passed the kitchen window she noticed something on the porch out of the corner of her sleepy eyes. To her delight, a closer look revealed what appeared to be a dog at her front door. Was this a dream?

Wiping the sleep from her eyes she opened the door and there, staring up at her was an adorable, basset hound-beagle mix puppy. Pat's husband advised her to leave it alone so it would return to its home. Well, two days of ignoring did not dissuade the orphan, so the couple finally fed the hungry hound.

Two weeks of searching the newspapers and grocery store bulletin boards and calling the animal control and police dispatch daily netted no owner. By now both husband and wife were smitten by the four-legged bundle of love and they welcomed her into their home and their family.

When she was truly willing to give up what she had waited her entire life for,

Pat's prayer was answered. Rosie, as the dog is known, has become a special blessing for the couple and has filled their lives with years of love.

Another concept that uses the prayer principle is the use of affirmations. Outside the discipline of meditation, an affirmation becomes a positive statement affirming what we want for our lives. An appropriate affirmation for the purpose of finding the right pet could be, "I am attracting the ideal pet into my life." Such an affirmation could be written on note cards and posted in strategic locations to act as a reminder of what we want.

As with prayer and meditation, simply repeating a phrase over and over is not likely to benefit us. The words are used purely to stir up a feeling. Our goal is to maintain an expectancy that our dream pet is on its way into our lives; in fact, it is already here.

Synchronicity

Synchronistic events are experiences that involve meaningful coincidences. Seemingly unrelated occurrences come together in a way that catches our attention. For example, a few months ago I awoke in the morning with an image from a dream. All I could remember was the name Magellan. It had no meaning for me at the time so it was quickly pushed to the back of my mind and all but forgotten. That evening, there was a news story about a car show in California. Dealers were showcasing their latest models. The story highlighted a new car called the Magellan. What a strange name for a car. I immediately remembered the image in my dream and felt the happenstance was a sign to look more closely at that dream symbol.

Such synchronicities acknowledge that we live in an orderly universe that is governed by immutable laws and where everything that happens has a purpose. Our Creator is intimately involved in our lives. Creation did not stop with Adam and Eve but is an ongoing event.

In fact, we are co-creators of our world and our experiences. Every choice we make, every word we say, every deed we do, and every thought we consider will have its effects on our future experiences. It may be that we will not fully appreciate the cause of certain experiences in this lifetime. Nevertheless, everything happens for a reason. This does not mean that bad things only happen to bad people and vice versa. There are more factors at play in the universe than we will ever understand. Of course, we will never understand the meaning of any of life's events if we don't look for it.

Once we acknowledge that life is meaningful we are left to make sense of it all. I have found that the more I connect with the Divine through meditation, prayer, and dream study, the more I recognize the significance of what is going on in my life. There is value in engaging fully—holistically—in all aspects of life.

So, just what does all this have to do with finding a compatible pet? In a synchronistic world, it is more than just a coincidence that a stray wandered up to your door or that your co-worker mentioned seeing a litter of cocker spaniel puppies for sale on her way to work when that was just the pet you were considering. At the same time, honoring synchronicity does not necessarily mean taking in every stray that you come across. It does not mean jumping into any and every situation that seems to present itself. Observation and analysis of synchronistic events is just another spiritual tool—like prayer, meditation, and dream work—to help with life decisions. A holistic approach to choosing the right pet honors all of these as well as intellectual factors.

There certainly is a lot to keep in mind when it comes to finding a pet. And here all along you thought the biggest decision was whether to take the black one or the gray one. No doubt, if you want a pet, you can find one even without putting much thought or effort into it. However, this book is not about just finding and caring for a pet. It is about consciously entering into and maintaining a meaningful relationship with an individual of another species. This is going to take some effort.

Intention is everything. What you hold in your heart affects your actions and both affect your circumstances and the lessons you are presented with. The universe picks up your thoughts and actions and reflects them back to you. Unselfish, caring intentions will help you get the relationship off on the right foot.

Your intentions and feelings are not only a means of communication with the Divine; they are also picked up by your animal companion. This is an important fact to remember when it comes to communicating with your animal friends.

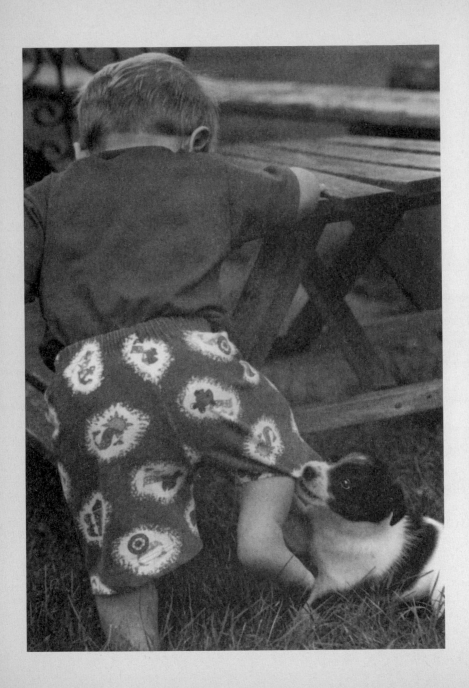

CHAPTER

3

ANIMAL COMMUNICATION

(Q) Could a life reading be obtained through these sources for
Aunt [268]'s little dog Mona?
(A) May be. As to *what* it may be is different! It may not be under-
stood, unless you learn dog language!   406-1

t first, the above quote sounds like a joking response. How ri-
diculous to expect someone to "learn dog language." Cayce apparently did not want to give a life reading for a dog, so he
made a sarcastic remark to silence the request. On the other hand, a
thoughtful examination of the concept of interspecies communication
reveals the truth of this idea. In order to have meaningful communication we do need to look at things from the animal's perspective.

Communication is an exchange of information. It involves whatever it takes to have one's thoughts understood by another. An idea must be formulated, transmitted, received, and interpreted. This process is complicated enough between two members of the same species who speak the same language. The task becomes even more difficult when the exchange of information is attempted between two very different types of beings with different languages, different modes of communication, different priorities, different cultures, and different spiritual purposes.

An exchange of ideas is the cornerstone of any relationship. It is paramount for us to communicate effectively with our animal friends in order to establish and maintain the pet connection. Our culture tends to look at communication with animals as a one-way street. We command them to follow our directions and bow to our wills. However, true communication involves give and take. To build a relationship we must observe and listen to our pets and strive to understand their distinctive natures.

Levels of Communication

There are many ways for people to get their messages across. We wave hello or good-bye. We put our hands on our hips out of anger and over our faces with embarrassment. We tell a joke with a smile and a wink. We bow our heads in prayer.

However, as humans we consider that we are mostly verbal communicators. We say what we mean. At critical times we choose our words wisely. Yet, as important as our words are at conveying our meaning, studies have shown that when speaking face to face, 55 percent of the message that is received is gleaned from body language. An additional 38 percent of the meaning is derived from voice inflection. That doesn't leave much for those carefully chosen words. On the phone, 86 percent of the message is determined not from what is said but rather how it is said.

Much of our body language is sent and received subconsciously. Sally didn't mean to give away her true feelings by her stiff posture, and Bob didn't notice it on the conscious level, he just knew something wasn't right.

Furthermore, humans communicate on a soul level. Most people have had the experience of walking into a room and feeling the stress. Sometimes the tension is so thick you can cut it with a knife. Many of us have also had feelings or intuitions about people we have just met. Psychic communication is more common than we realize.

Animals, too, correspond on many levels simultaneously. Scent is a major form of communication for them as is body language. The meow of the cat and the bark of the dog also testify to the existence of at least a limited animal oral language. Although they cannot form words, dogs and cats usually get their messages across by how they vocalize. Perhaps pets also communicate on a psychic level as we do.

Communicating with pets intuitively does appear to be possible, even for the novice. However, knowing visual cues for communication is much more important because animal body language is more obvious to us than their mental messages. Plus, we often misinterpret the objective of animal language. Later we will look at the use of intuition in conversing with our pets, but first let's explore how animals communicate on the physical level so we can read their body language and avoid miscommunication.

Animal Sense

Because communication on the physical level depends on the five senses, it is extremely important to understand just how different we are from our animal companions in the way we experience the world around us.

From a scientific standpoint, it is impossible for us to know exactly what animals see, hear, smell, taste, and feel. We know quite a bit about the various sense organs of animals. This tells us what stimuli they take in, but how an animal interprets this sensory data is determined by the creature's mind. On the physical level we can examine an animal's brain, but we have yet to dissect a mind.

Smell

Because the area of the brain related to the sense of smell dominates the feline and canine craniums, scientists have determined that the most dominant sense for our companion animals is the sense of smell. This idea is further supported by the fact that dogs and cats have many more cells in their sinus cavities that detect odors than people do. For example, cats have hundreds of millions of these scent–sensitive cells while people have only five million.

Cats even have an extra gland called the vomero–nasal or Jacobson's organ located behind their front teeth, to further aid their sense of smell. Have you ever witnessed your cat raise her head slightly, lift her upper lip and open her mouth a little? The posture is often accompanied by a look of intense concentration and a flicking of the tongue inside the mouth. This strange behavior is known as the Flehman response and indicates that the cat is transmitting scent material to her Jacobson's organ and gaining extra information about her environment.

It is difficult for us to consider living in a world where odors rule. Can you imagine what our world would "look" like if our sense of smell was several times stronger than our eyesight? We need to open our minds to a different way of seeing things if we ever hope to understand our pets. In their world, odors play a major role in communication.

Have you ever seen a hound track a rabbit? Can you imagine following the scent of a running rabbit? What a keen nose he must have. Have you ever seen two kitty friends fight like strangers after one of them returns from the veterinarian's office? The cat that remained at home is so aware of the odors that his friend has picked up at the clinic that he does not recognize his companion. Our pets mark their territory with scent as well. This is a powerful form of communication that we are usually unaware of due to our inferior sense of smell.

Vision

There are many differences in visual perception between pets and people as well. From the anatomy of the eyes of dogs and cats, it is clear that they see things differently than we do. One factor to explore is visual acuity or the ability to distinguish the fine details of objects.

The central 25 percent of the retinas of the dog's eye (the most important part for vision) is predominated by light–gathering rod cells. In humans, this visual center of the eye has mostly color–seeing cone cells. This allows animals to see better (have better visual acuity) in the dark than we do. Animals also have a reflective area in their retinas, called the tapetum, which further augments their night vision. In fact, the cat eye is six times more sensitive to light than the human eye. It appears that the dog's eye is slightly less sensitive than that of the cat.

At the same time, in normal daylight humans have better vision than pets do. A major reason for this is that the human optic nerve has 1.2 million fibers while that of the dog has only 167,000 and the cat's has between 116,000 and 165,000. Scientific studies estimate that the average dog has about twenty/seventy–five vision. This means that from twenty feet away, dogs can only begin to distinguish the details of an object that a person can see from seventy–five feet away. There is also an indication that some dogs become nearsighted (can only see close up) as they age.

Our pets' ability to see in dim light comes at the expense of their color vision. Early studies indicated that dogs are color blind but more recent research has clarified this issue. Finding fewer cones cells in the central retina indicates that they see colors less vividly. Dogs also have only two types of cones while people have three. This means that while people can sense all the colors in the visual spectrum, dogs cannot distinguish between green, yellow, orange, and red and cannot tell greenish–blue from gray.

Because of how the canine eyes are positioned on the head, dogs have better peripheral vision than we do. However, this ocular placement means that dogs have a lesser degree of binocular overlap. To translate, less of their field of view has depth perception compared to ours.

We should also take into consideration how the relative height of our pets affects their perception. Sometimes we take our ability to see over things for granted. For instance, while walking a toy poodle through a crowd of people, the owner can see over and above at least some of the pedestrians. At the same time, the pitiful pooch is struggling through a forest of moving legs and stepping shoes. Of course the smaller stature may come in handy for hiding under the bed after raiding the cat's food.

In the dark of night, animals are visually aware of their surroundings. We can't hold a candle to their night vision. Yet in the light of day, we see colors and details more vividly. We have a wider area of depth perception, but they have better peripheral vision. What effect do these dissimilarities in vision play in our companions' abilities to receive visual cues of communication?

Hearing

The canine and feline sense of hearing is different than ours as well. They pick up a wider range of pitches. The pitch of a tone is its frequency which is measured in cycles per second or hertz. The human ear can detect pitches ranging from sixty to 20,000 hertz. We hear best at the range of 2,000 to 4,000 hertz.

Our pets can pick up both higher and lower frequencies than we can. A dog's ear can detect frequencies of thirty hertz to 48,000 hertz. The cat can hear pitches from thirty to a whopping 95,000 hertz. So dogs can hear about an octave higher than we can and cats can hear an octave and a half above that. Both dogs and cats hear best at frequencies of 4,000 to 8,000 hertz, well above our optimal range.

So remember that animals are not little people. Although our furry companions are equipped with the same sense organs we are, they experience their surroundings much differently than we do. We may share the same environment but live in totally different universes. Due to the importance of the five senses to communication, the difference in physical sensory perception between animals and people must be remembered when considering interspecies communication.

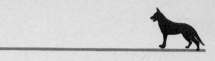

The Domestication Effect

Much of what our companion animals are today is a result of cohabitating with humans for tens of thousands of years. This applies to behavioral as well as physical attributes. The process of domestication involves the selective breeding of particular individuals for desired traits. For example, a friendly pet is much more likely to result from the union of two friendly animals than it is from the breeding of two nasty ones. Coincidentally, most of the behaviors that people find desirable such as friendliness, subordination, the propensity to vocalize, and trainability are all infantile animal behaviors. So, over the millennia, humans have bred and cared for animals who display immature behaviors as adults.

As a result of domestication many of out pets' communication behaviors are infantile when compared to those of their wild counterparts. A case in point is the fact that domestic cats vocalize. Wild species of cats vocalize as kits but lose that tendency as adults. Our adult cats meow because this juvenile behavior has been fostered by human intervention. We like animals that "talk" to us, so vocal cats have received preferential treatment. Many other behaviors of pets are carryovers from infantile interactions that young animals have with their parents. Domestic dogs and cats are genetically programmed to remain somewhat immature and often naturally accept their human caregivers as surrogate parents.

In spite of human intervention, cats and dogs have also retained their own distinctive cultures and modes of communication. Cats, dogs, and humans have developed individually over millions of years before our strands in the web of life became intertwined. Animals have well-ingrained instincts as well as social mores that have not succumbed to the will of their "masters." Let's explore some basics of objective animal communication.

Doggie Dialogue

As with humans, canines too converse with many modalities. In general it is necessary to be aware of the dog's entire display to understand his meaning. Looking at just the ears or just the tail is likely to be misleading. Without looking at the entire body it is difficult to make heads or tails of what he is saying. We'll first look at some broad guidelines about specific canine gestures; then we'll look at how dogs send particular messages.

Before embarking on this discussion, let's briefly look at a peculiar canine social trend. Canines are pack animals. In the wild, a pack functions as a team. In such instances it is very important that all the team members know their places. So dogs instinctively set up a pecking order among those they are living with. The hierarchy of command is so important that dominance versus submission often dominates the topic of discussion between dogs. Not every dog wants to be top dog but they all do want to know that there is a leader of the pack.

Dogs are not necessarily dominant or submissive by nature. The degree of dominance a particular canine displays is dependent on his circumstances and the group he is with. So dominance is a relative term. Although some dogs certainly have more overbearing tendencies than others, any dog may become dominant or submissive given the right circumstances.

Canine Body Language

When with others, a dog asserts his dominant stature with a set display. He stands tall with his head and tail held high and ears erect and forward. He may put a paw on the other dog's shoulders to emphasize his dominance. Although it is usually thought of as a sexual behavior, dogs often mount one another to express their dominance. This behavior may be carried out by either males or females, even pets that have been "fixed." When a dog mounts a person's leg it is not a sign of misplaced affection but rather a clear indication of disrespect.

So when one dog wants to challenge another and say, "I'm better than you," he gets over, above, and on top of his acquaintance. That is the same message we send to a dog when we bend over the top of them to give them a hug. We think of it as a sign of affection, but a dog that does not know us well may take it as a personal affront. A less aggressive salutation involves crouching down to the dog's level in front of him and letting him approach us.

An aggressive dog leans forward with his tail and ears up and forward. His hackles—the hair over his shoulders—may be bristled and he might even stand on his toes all in an attempt to appear larger and more formidable. The tail may be bristled and it will either be still or wagging in short, fast strokes. This posture is often accompanied by a snarl and a growl. The topper is that his eyes will lock yours in a bone-chilling stare as if to say, "You want a piece of this?" If you maintain face-to-face eye contact, he will read your response to be, "Bring it on, Bucko!" and you may soon find yourself in a scrap.

A submissive dog tries to make himself look smaller. In doing so he is saying, "Don't worry about me, I'm no threat to you." To make his point the meek canine will cower with his head lowered and ears back and down. He will avoid challenging eye contact. He will tuck his tail and may make pawing motions with his front paws. In extreme submission he may roll on his back and even dribble a little urine. Keep in mind that not all submissive behavior denotes fear. It can also be a sign of respect and trust.

A happy dog greets his caregiver with a bounding gait, wildly wagging tail, and panting, ear-to-ear, dog smile. Often as he nears his beloved guardian he will crouch, lower his ears, and wag his tail as a show of respect and submission. When he licks a person's face, it is another sign of the animal's lower status borrowed from his puppy days when he licked his mother's face in like manner.

When he's feeling playful a dog will often lower his chest to the ground and leave his rear end and wagging tail sticking up. His ears are alert and forward and he may give a high-pitched "yip." This posture is called the play bow and is a sure sign that Bowser is ready for some fun. In both of these situations the canine's eyes are relaxed and he will often look away or lower his gaze in deference.

The canine ear comes in many shapes and sizes. Droopy–eared dogs can only move the bases of their ears, so the gesticulations are not as dramatic as those of their pointy–eared brethren. When a dog's ears are erect and forward, the animal is alert, but this may be a friendly aware-ness or an aggressive preparedness. When a dog holds his ears down and back it can be a sign of submission, anxiety, or fearfulness. It is important to realize that a fearful dog can become just as aggressive as a dominant dog. You need to look at the entire package to get the mes-sage.

The tail of the dog is equally tricky to decipher. In fact, in some breeds of dogs, the tail is downright hard to detect. For example, Pugs, with their tightly wound pig tails, usually end up wagging their entire bod-ies to let their caregivers know they are happy. Speaking of tail wag-ging, we are all familiar with the fact that dogs wag their tails when they are happy and playful. However, they also wag their tails when they are feeling aggressive. A dog with a wagging tail is not necessarily inviting you to approach.

Interestingly, dogs tend not to wag their tails at all when they are alone. Even when playing happily, the solitary canine's tail is inclined to be dormant. So the tail wag seems to be a purposeful, communication skill. Other generalizations about the tail are that if it is held high the pet may be alert and interested or assertive and aggressive. If the tail is tucked the dog is either respectful, submissive, or fearful. Again, be cau-tious of the fearfully aggressive canine.

Dogs have other peculiar gestures as well. For us, yawning is a sign of boredom. However, when a dog yawns it usually means he is anxious and stressed. Some dogs flick their tongues up and lick their noses re-peatedly when feeling uneasy. Often a dog nudges his caregiver with his nose to beg for attention. Leaning on you is sometimes another ploy for attention but it can also be an assertive dog's way of expanding his personal space at your expense. Some dogs, especially Golden Retriev-ers, actually draw their lips back in a smile, baring their teeth when they are feeling happy and friendly. This display can look startlingly like a snarl if you do not read the rest of the body language.

Canine Vocalization

The dog's vocal abilities are narrow compared to ours. A bark can mean many things depending on how it is delivered. The spectrum ranges from the harsh, assertive, aggressive bark to the light "play with me" woof. While most dogs bark to communicate something specific, others do it out of habit or out of boredom.

Howling is the canine way of communicating with each other over long distances. A wimpy whine can mean the dog wants attention or it may indicate fear, stress, or submissiveness. A growl is usually a warning although some pups growl during play and mean nothing by it.

Feline Lingo

In order to understand our feline friends we must understand their natures. Cats have been labeled as being antisocial. Nothing could be further from the truth. Any cat lover will tell you that most cats love to interact with each other and their human housemates. The reason that cats have gotten their asocial reputation is that they have a different social structure than humans or even dogs.

Both humans and dogs are basically pack animals and their social structures are based on team work. Cats, on the other hand, developed from an independent species of felines. Instead of issues of hierarchy dominating their conversations, cats are more concerned about territory. So, as we shall see, felines spend a lot of time "discussing" exactly what belongs to whom.

Feline Vocalization

The feline vocal repertory is limited but effective. On the unpleasant end of the spectrum we have the raspy, drawn out, "yowling" of a cornered cat. This noise signifies fear but is accompanied by the threat that if the approach is continued, there will be violent consequences. If pressed further, the threatened feline will usually give its last warning consisting of hissing and spitting. If this danger signal goes unheeded, the cat is likely to lash out, tooth and nail.

It is amazing the respect that a hissing cat can command. This relatively diminutive utterance can strike fear into the heart of even a large canine aggressor. Apparently it's not what you say but how you say it that is important in the animal kingdom, too. I guess it is true that if you want to get someone's attention, just whisper.

The simple cat meow takes on many meanings depending on voice inflection and other non-verbal cues. There is the demanding "I want food!" meow directed at the caregiver when the food bowl is empty. This is usually accompanied by obvious gestures toward the deficient food receptacle or the insistent clawing of the owner's leg. (Cats never beg!) The observant cat fancier will eventually detect other variations on the meow. There are complaining meows, anxious meows, and the ever popular "pet me!" meows.

Cats sometimes make a sound described as a rising trill. This is the same noise a mother cat makes to greet and gather her kittens. Cats will sometimes use this greeting to welcome their owners home after their absence. Feline vocabulary also includes a chirping sound that they sometimes mutter while intently watching small critters from opposite sides of the window pane. It is almost as if they are saying, "Come here little birdie."

By far the most sought after feline intonation is the low, soft, vibratory purr. Purring originates in kittenhood. Nursing kittens make this sound to let their mother know that all is well and the milk is flowing. In adulthood, cats often purr when they are content and comfortable. They seem to be saying, "I'm feeling friendly." However, cats also sometimes purr when they are injured or feel threatened. Occasionally my feline patients purr while on my office exam table, and I know it is not because they are having fun. In such cases, the purr may be an attempt to placate any possible threat while in a vulnerable state. They are probably saying, "I'm friendly, don't hurt me."

Just a side note about purring; it is possible that purring has more than communication value in the cat. Recent research by the Fauna Communications Research Institute in Hillsborough, North Carolina, studied the purrs of both domestic and wild felines. They found that the dominant frequencies of the purrs for three species were exactly twenty-five Hz or fifty Hz. These frequencies have been shown in other studies to be effective for promoting bone growth and repair. Perhaps purring is the cat's way of tapping into vibrational healing. It is true that cat's bones heal faster than dog's and that dogs are much more prone to arthritis.

The Eyes Have It

Cats seem to communicate a lot to each other through the use of their eyes. I have a cat that can shoot a glance across a room that makes any approaching feline reverse direction. The eyes are said to be the windows of the soul. Your cat's pupils can give away her emotional state. When the pupils are dilated, it means she is excited. Now this excitement may take two basic forms. She may be pleasantly excited, as when her food bowl is being filled, or she may be aroused due to the fear of a threatening situation. The opposite case is that of the fearless, dominant, aggressive cat. Such an animal will often have pupils that are contracted into thin slits. Of course, both the fearless and fearful cat can be equally dangerous.

Even the degree of opening or closing of the eyelids speaks loudly about how a cat is feeling. Wide-open eyelids signify an alert cat in an uncertain situation. A cat who is perfectly content peers out of half-opened eyes. Cats obviously close their eyes completely when they are sleeping. They also shut their eyes as a sign of submission when the battle with another cat is lost. The loser will turn away from the aggressor and close her eyes both to protect these fragile organs and to appease the antagonist.

Love-struck humans gaze longingly into each other's eyes for hours on end. However, staring for prolonged a period directly into your cat's eyes sends a different signal. Locking eyes means aggression to your feline friend. This cultural difference in nonverbal communication can lead to misunderstandings.

Feline Body Language

If you watch your cat closely, you will notice how certain postures relate to her moods. Ear position is an obvious place to start. In the typical, relaxed kitty the ear openings face forward and somewhat to the sides. When the ears are erect and pointing forward it means the cat is excited and alert. An agitated feline's ears will tend to twitch. When on the defensive, the cat holds her ears flattened tight against her head. Finally, if the ears are rotated back but not fully flattened so the backs of the ears are visible from the front, you are looking at an aggressive cat in attack mode.

Cats also "talk" with a certain sign language using their tails. Watch your cat closely and see if you can read the tail she tells. When the tail curves down then up at the tip, it means she is content. A raised curving tail signifies the cat is beginning to pay attention to something. If the tail is straight up with the tip bent, the kitty is interested and in a friendly mood but with some reservations. When your cat greets you with no reservations, her tail is fully erect. When a cat tucks her tail, she is signaling defeat and submission. When a cat wags her tail violently from side to side, you can bet she is angry.

A bristled tail indicates the fight or flight response. Animals often use the fluffing technique to appear bigger and to scare off their adversary. Cats augment this display by hunching their backs and turning sideways to further increase their apparent size. If the fluffed-up tail is held down, the cat is in defensive mode; if it is straight up, the cat is on the offensive.

There are other uniquely feline gestures that are sometimes misunderstood. Some cats like to jump up on their caregiver's lap and knead away with their front feet like a miniature masseuse. This appears to be another behavior that is carried on from kittenhood. While nursing kittens purr to reassure their mother, they also knead at her underside to help stimulate the flow of milk. When an adult cat does this, it seems to mean that she is happy, comfortable, and feeling well cared for.

Cats often rub up against the legs of their caregivers when greeting them. Contrary to popular belief, this is not an attempt to trip the humans. Rather, the behavior is a way of marking the person with scent while at the same time gathering chemical information. Cats have scent glands on their temples, inner lips, and at the base of their tails. While mouthing, rubbing, and entwining your legs, your cat is marking and claiming you. After rubbing its entire body against you, your cat may then lick her flank to pick up scent data from you. This exchange is a valuable form of communication for your cat and a source of endearment for you.

One not–so–endearing communication behavior of cats is territorial marking. This often takes two forms. The most obvious way that cats mark their property is by spraying urine. Urinating outside the litter box is sometimes a kitty's way of letting her caregiver know that she is feeling insecure. Another way for cats to mark their territory is by scratching vertical objects. Cats have scent glands in their paws. When a cat scratches the furniture, drapery, or walls, it is saying, "Private property, keep out." These last two problematic kitty communication techniques will be discussed more thoroughly in the next chapter, which deals with animal behavior modification.

It takes time and careful observation to read and understand some of the subtleties of animal body language. Unwitting humans often misconstrue the signs the animal sends. We also sometimes send erroneous messages to our animals through our improper gestures. Animal body language is extremely reliable. Once you understand how to interpret the language, what you see is what you get. Anyone who pays attention can pick up on their pet's communication and thus avoid misunderstandings.

For their part, animals do not understand English or any other human language. Pets can be trained to respond to certain words or short phrases, but it does no good to lecture a dog on the pros and cons of chewing your new shoes. If your pet does pick up on your meaning at times, it is because she has learned to understand the meaning of your body language and tone of voice. Or perhaps sometimes, when the conditions are right, your pet also can read your thoughts.

Intuitive Pet Communication

Telepathic animal communication is simply a transfer of information and/or feelings from one being to another. It involves tapping into the field of information and energy that, according to quantum physics, pervades the universe. The ability to communicate in this way is not supernatural. On the contrary, it is quite natural. We all have this talent, and with practice we can develop it further.

Just as we can learn a lot by watching our pets' body language, it can be equally rewarding to approach our companion animals from the perspective of thought transmission. Communicating intuitively requires the refinement of certain skills. Whereas physical exchange depends on paying attention to our five senses, communicating at the intuitive level relies on closely observing our inner senses.

In order to get a deeper perspective on telepathic animal communication, I have enlisted the help of several professionals in this area. I have interviewed animal intuitives in whose skills I am confident. I am offering more than one view because we are each different in the ways that we send, receive, and interpret intuitive information. The broader the range of insight into this mysterious skill, the more likely each reader is to connect with some concept that is put forth.

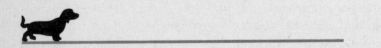

Introducing Our Animal Communicators

Dr. Agnes Thomas—I have always been drawn to animals ever since I was a pre-schooler. My grandmother had a farm and there were lots of animals I grew to know and appreciate. I guess the real interest began when Walt Disney made us see animals as beings instead of food or livestock used as beasts of burden. I wondered if my grandmother's barnyard beings talked to each other, formed attachments and relationships, and most of all, if they loved me back. Even at that early age, I "knew" I was loved and welcome among them.

In kindergarten, my grandmother gave me a kitten. I remember being overwhelmed by the unconditional love being extended to me by the kitten. I believed that kitty understood that I felt the same way about her, without thinking in terms of two-way communication at that time. When she got lost, I searched for her up and down the streets after school, even in deep snow. I never found her, but the bond between us remained even into high school.

College was an opportunity to study the human psyche. I chose to specialize in physiological psychology because I could also work with animals. I studied the brain, mind, and learning abilities of laboratory animals, such as rats, mice, hamsters, and guinea pigs. Studies of this kind are used to make inferences about how humans think and feel.

It was only natural to continue to investigate the mind of human and nonhuman beings. During the illness of one of my cats, I came in contact with an animal communicator, who talked to the cat directly, and I found her communications helpful and fascinating. It was a next logical step in my career to combine psychological counseling with communications with both human and nonhuman beings.

I went around the country to study with people who knew how to communicate with animals telepathically, and acquired the skill. Animal communication is a real eye-opener. I had no idea there was so much loveliness in all life around me.

Betsy Crouse—I've been fascinated with animals my whole life and have worked with them in many capacities. We always had many animals in the house growing up, and I brought home every lost, sick, and baby animal I came across for years. I studied biology in college and several years after that studied and became certified to teach therapeutic horseback riding. I began to study metaphysics in my mid-twenties, and have continued to do so for the past twenty years.

Always, my interest in deepening my relationship with the animals in my life grew. I studied and experimented with different training approaches, especially drawn to teaching with positive reinforcement. I took several workshops with Linda Tellington-Jones, learning and utilizing her T-Touch methods. When I was twenty-five, I read a book titled *Kinship With All Life,* by J. Allen Boone, and listened to a cassette tape by Penelope Smith, a pioneer in the field of interspecies telepathic communication. Those two experiences reopened a door within me. The idea of communication with animals on the mental/emotional level did not seem far out to me; instead, it felt like I was being reminded of what I'd known and forgotten.

From that time onward, I began to explore this area actively. Learning and practicing meditation helped me develop the ability to quiet my own mind. In time, I began to experience clearer mental/emotional impressions when I was working with animals. I experimented with sending messages on this level, also, and had experiences that made it abundantly clear to me that the animals were receiving those messages. I began to think about becoming involved with communication work with others and took advanced training with Penelope Smith.

The work I do has evolved into a combination of training/behavioral/communication work, with a strong emphasis on helping people communicate better with their own animals. I recommend Bach flower remedies in some cases, and do some energetic healing work. I am moving in the direction of focusing on integrating positive reinforcement training methods with telepathic sending skills, which I feel allows me to offer something of practical use to a wide group of animal lovers and their animal friends.

Renee Takacs—I am a full-time, intuitive consultant with twelve years of experience conducting intuitive consultations for both people and pets. I facilitate workshops and forums for intuition development. My corporate and nonprofit audiences have included Aetna U.S. Healthcare, Conrail, Columbia Gas of Pennsylvania, Howard Hanna Real Estate, the Western Pennsylvania Humane Society, Animal Rescue League, Keystone Canine Club, and the Collie Frolic, among many others.

The Association for Research and Enlightenment and its members, of which I am one, continue to be a wonderfully supportive resource. In 2000, I felt quite humbled when the A.R.E. selected me from an extensive pool of intuitives to serve on the psychic panel during the annual Edgar Cayce Legacy week.

With the intent to educate the public on the purpose and value of intuition, I began to write articles about my animal readings. Rodale Press's *Pets, Part of the Family* magazine, May/June 2000, featured my article, "The Apple Answer to a Frightened Pet." The radio and television appearances I have made have allowed me to reach a broader audience than I thought possible when I first started to consult. I've always desired to help people develop their own intuition. Since 1997 I've hosted a weekly Intuitive Circle Night. This forum welcomes individuals who are interested in developing their intuition in a spiritually sound environment.

My education includes a master's degree in transpersonal studies from Atlantic University, Virginia Beach, Virginia (1996), and a B.S.B.A. from Robert Morris College, Pittsburgh, Pennsylvania (1981). In 1995, by invitation from Jeffrey Mishlove of the Intuition Network and PBS's "Thinking Allowed" series, I presented the findings of my original, master's thesis research in the field of intuitive consulting for business leaders at the international intuition conference in Denver, Colorado.

Studies which I feel have contributed to my sensitivity have included the various healing modalities, such as Therapeutic Touch and reiki, and a brief but meaningful exposure to the martial art aikido. However, the greatest experience that has contributed to my sensitivity is yoga. I've been a yoga instructor for over a dozen years. Yoga served as a major influence in developing my intuition.

The Questions Please

In an attempt to tap the knowledge of these animal communicators and to afford ease of comparison, I have asked each of these professionals the same questions. Here are those questions and each animal communicator's response.

What got you started on your path as an animal communicator?

Dr. Agnes Thomas—One of my cats developed a brain tumor and I consulted an animal communicator in order to help him. When I spoke to my cat, I was deeply touched because he called me "mommy." Later in the conversation, I asked him if he was going to live. He answered, "I am not concerned with my physical life, only my spiritual life." I asked if he realized how much the veterinarians and staff loved him. He said, "Mommy, I was supposed to do that. That was my mission." His mission? That told me that animals are capable of deductive reasoning, and also of planning and carrying out specific and intentional acts of kindness.

The communicator validated his responses and gave examples of other acts of kindness given to humans by animals. As a psychologist, I was fascinated and wanted to learn much more from animals. Because I am interested in the mind and brain, I looked into animal communication further.

Betsy Crouse—Primarily, my deep desire to better understand the animals in my life, and to "do right" in my interactions with them. It has been clear to me for a very long time that our limited ability to understand animals creates difficulties for them. As children, we are not encouraged to retain a sensitive and active imagination. We lose our ability to really empathize with animals as we grow up in Western culture, becoming immersed in a human perspective and experience.

From there, we tend to project positive and negative human attributes onto animals, using those projections as a foundation for our conclusions about animals' needs, wants, and abilities, and their willingness, or lack thereof, to cooperate with us. This is a huge injustice, and sets them up to fail in our world. Failure to abide by our rules carries very stiff penalties for animals, sometimes as extreme as death.

I am passionate about helping human beings better understand that, for all their qualities which we relate to and/or are charmed by, animals are intensely unlike us in fundamental ways that differ from species to species. We must strive to perceive non-humans as they truly are, not as we assume them to be. Reawakening my own sensitivity to more subtle levels of communication, and working to always strengthen the clarity of that level of perception, is at the heart of my passion to contribute in this area of human-animal relationships.

Also, I am simply and profoundly fascinated with the natural world, and with animals in particular. And I'm fascinated with the "worlds-beyond–our–world," or the nonphysical aspects and layers and dimensions that exist beyond our current sensory perceptions.

Renee Takacs—My initial start as an animal communicator was my wish as a child to talk to the animals like the movies that inspired me, *Dr. Doolittle* and many of the Disney movies. While growing up I spent most of my time in the woods observing the little animals that scampered by wondering, what were they thinking? Where did they live? Did they have sisters or a family like I had? Cats, dogs, horses, and cows surrounded our property where I grew up. Everyday barnyard scents and sounds drifted through our yard from the neighbor's farm. The farm's excess of cats, along with our family dog, became my playmates.

My professional start as an animal communicator began after seven years as an intuitive consultant doing readings for people. One afternoon I was invited to do a reading for a dog! I was at a client's home preparing to leave when fate ignited the spark within me. My client teased me about reading for her family dog, a collie shepherd mixed breed. Acting on the impulse, I asked, "Do you mind if I try?" The next thing I knew I was receiving impressions about where he liked to sleep, which was in the back bedroom with a blanket over his head. He also told me he was missing his bacon treat. My client's boyfriend's jaw dropped. The boyfriend explained that for many weeks that bacon treat had been on the grocery list and everyone kept forgetting to pick it up!

What form does the communication take for you?

Dr. Agnes Thomas—Communication takes different forms for different people, and sometimes several forms for one communicator. Mine is primarily visual. However, since I have a medical background, I always ask the animal how their health is. They show me the inside of their body, and often send sensations of pain or illness to me, which I receive through the gut. Depending on the problem, sometimes they will also send me an auditory communication, or even a special taste, which I receive through the mouth. Sometimes it takes the form of a combination of all of these.

The message itself, is a composite of all the animal sees, hears, smells, tastes, feels, and its desires at any given moment in time. It is received as a complete impression by the communicator. It has to be filtered through the communicator's own brain and be translated into language or pictures according to how much the communicator has in their own brains. For example, if my sister asks an animal how he feels, he may say "I have a stomach ache." The same message sent to me, would consist of the animal showing me his alimentary tract, any blockages, pain, or growths associated with the stomach ache.

To send communications to an animal I talk to the person and follow their heart connection to the animal (over the phone). Once I locate the animal, I validate their location in the home by describing where the dog/cat is sitting, standing, or whatever. Once I am sure I have the right pet, then I generally send them a message by concentrating on talking to them as if we were only two or three feet apart. The first time I connect requires going into an altered state to find the animal. Once this is accomplished, I merely need to think of the animal to connect.

Betsy Crouse—It varies quite a lot for me. When sending communication, I use a range of things to help make myself clear. I use images, feelings, and imagined bodily sensations to help convey information. I will often put myself, in my imagination, in the place of the animal I'm connecting with, to help communicate about things like physical orientation and body movement. I use words, also, as a means to focus my intention, images, and feelings. Sometimes I talk out loud, sometimes silently, depending on which brings better clarity to my focus.

When receiving communication, I usually experience specific emotional feelings, and sometimes specific images, and/or imagined sounds, smells, or other sensory impressions. Sometimes words are included, although I believe this is a "translation" of my own consciousness, which may happen so rapidly it seems as if the animal is communicating in English. Other times I have the experience of getting what seems like a "package" of information, which may then take several minutes to sort out into linear expression.

Renee Takacs—The communication begins when I shift into a state of soft, loving receptivity and ask for permission from the animal to speak with him/her. I set my mental intention to receive information that the pet wants to relay or that the pet's person needs to know or would find most helpful knowing at the time. Stating the intent instantly connects me with the animal, whether the animal is here or in spirit. Love is the key that opens communication and hearts.

I receive either a feeling from the animal that feels welcoming or I sometimes hear words as the animal responds, such as "Hi" or "I'm ready," or "I've been waiting for you," as though the animal knew even before I did that we were going to speak.

I ask the animal, "Is there anything you want to tell me?" and the conversation begins. I receive images, feel physical sensations, hear words, discern the emotional tone, smell what they smell, and hear what they hear.

How do you know that the information you are giving and receiving is coming from/going to the animal?

Dr. Agnes Thomas—It takes much practice and a good teacher in order for one to discern with clarity what is actually coming from the animal and what part may be coming from you—trying to figure out the answer. The best indicator that it is coming from the animal is the speed of the answer. You should receive the answer before the rest of the question is out of your mouth. It is mind-to-mind communication.

Betsy Crouse—I rely on a combination of my sense of focus, and the strength of my intention, to know that communication with an animal is "on track." If my mind wanders, if I'm overly aware of outside distractions, if I'm questioning the communication itself, if I'm planning my response while listening—I've lost contact.

The feeling I have when I'm clearly connected is very similar to the feeling when involved in an intense conversation with a human being who has my full attention and respect. When I am listening, I'm completely focused on my companion, giving myself over to really hearing them. When I'm talking, I'm doing my best to be clear and honest, to not send mixed messages, to be sensitive to the impact I may be having.

There are times when I am attempting to send or receive mental/emotional communication while under stress myself. An example is a time when my dog, Travis, was lost, and there have been other times when an animal friend has been ill or unhappy. At those times, my own stress may make it hard for me to be as clearly and quietly focused as I would like, and I simply do the best I can.

Whether in a stressful situation or not, I always ask for help with this level of communication; help in maintaining the highest level of integrity of which I am capable; help in truly understanding the animal I am connecting with.

Renee Takacs—I simply know. Setting the intent opens the door to that specific animal. Many of the impressions I receive are specific to the animal species and are different from people readings. For instance, with cats and dogs I see a lot of human feet and shoes, smell some really intense smells (not necessarily the feet!) and most of the time feel a more consistently pronounced feeling of devotion, love, and forgiveness than generally what I sense with people.

When I'm reading over the phone and have never met the animal, the pet's person often verifies the information I'm giving them about their pet with a tone of confirming surprise in their voice. If the reading is conducted in person, the animal often becomes quiet and calm. My client's have repeatedly commented from observation that their pet will turn his/her head directly toward me for a moment just when I'm telepathically asking their pet a specific question.

Lastly, I know for certain when I'm linked with an animal because the animal never asks, "When am I going to get rich?" or "When am I going to get married?!"

What tips do you have to help the typical caregiver to communicate with his/her pet?

Dr. Agnes Thomas—Animals know your intentions. They can hear your thoughts even though you cannot hear theirs. They think we are deaf. Pet owners should always talk to their pets as if they understand. Tell them when they are going to the vet, what will happen there, if they are going on vacation, how many days they will be gone, and things like who will take care of them while they are gone. This gives them a better sense of how to still maintain a connection with the pet owner while they are away. Pets keep their connection regardless of distance. Older pets have a harder time of keeping the bond, especially over very long distances, e.g., between New York and California. It saves them the anxiety associated with separation, and calms them. Separation anxiety can be severe, leading to terrible confusion for the pet, and resulting in such behaviors as inappropriate bowel and bladder eliminations.

All animals are here to help their persons with their spiritual journey. Most animals will tell you what their mission is if you ask.

Betsy Crouse—Slow down. Pay attention. Let go of agendas. Don't give mixed messages. Many of us who live very busy lives seldom make the time to truly slow down. And even when we do slow down physically, our minds and emotions often remain in a jumble. When it comes to communicating clearly with our animals (on any level), I feel that the first step is for us to learn to really and truly slow down and focus our attention.

Learning how to meditate is probably the single most helpful thing I would recommend in this regard. Meditation takes many, many forms, so don't think this has to mean sitting on a pillow contemplating your navel! Although sitting meditation is a powerful avenue to altering our state of consciousness, I think it is also one of the more difficult ways for a beginner to learn about meditating.

Altering our state of consciousness is exactly what is meant when we talk about learning to send and receive clear, focused communication on the mental/emotional level. We need to learn to step out of our fast-lane, left-brain chatter and into a state of mind and being that is quiet and focused.

Learning to pay attention to detail is paramount to broadening perception, in my opinion. We can start by paying attention to detail on the physical level. That is one of the reasons I love teaching people about positive reinforcement operant conditioning (PROC), or clicker training. Traditional training methods are mostly about telling animals what to do; PROC is all about learning to listen to your animals; asking them how much they do or don't understand, asking them if they are still with you as you make your way through a lesson with them. Learning to really observe and listen on this more familiar, physical level can help pave the way to deeper levels of listening.

Letting go of agendas is essential to successful communication with animals. It is especially needed for perception of mental/emotional messages, when we are learning to focus our attention in ways that are strange and unfamiliar, and working to develop skill with very subtle avenues of connection. Often, I think we already have a clear idea of how we want things to go in a situation with an animal friend, and our preconceptions get in the way of clear communication.

We may be impatient to move a situation along, we may be fearful of an undesired answer, we may be stuck in our own thoughts and emotions concerning certain circumstances. It's important to learn how to set aside agendas that are already coloring the outcome in an exchange of communication. This is more easily said than done, but simply becoming aware of what our agendas are is a powerful start.

Taking care not to send mixed messages is important in developing better sending skills. It is very common for people to be saying something different on the physical, mental, and emotional levels. Negative expectations, especially, cause problems. For example, consider what you are thinking and feeling (and therefore what mental/emotional messages you are sending) as you call a dog who has run away from you before, attempt to trim the nails of a cat who has bitten you for this in the past, or prepare to load a horse who has a reputation for being very difficult about trailers. In all those situations, you are most likely having thoughts and feelings that conflict directly with what you are asking of and wanting from your animal.

I would also strongly encourage people to imagine success. By this I mean imagining yourself having the kind of communication relationship you dream of with your animals. Imagine it in detail, and add to it as time goes by. Work to develop a richness of texture with this desired future that matches the level of detail and intimacy you can generate when imagining something very familiar. In so doing, you are setting the stage to draw to yourself the experiences and resources that will help you move in the direction of that future relationship you desire.

Renee Takacs—The first tip I offer is to believe that you can communicate with your pet. Choose a quiet time and place yourself in a loving, receptive mode. Set your intent, "I now desire to communicate with my pet." Ask your pet with a feeling tone of love from your heart, "Is there anything you want to tell me?" or "How are you?"

Trust the impressions you receive through inner feeling, hearing, seeing, memories, or even lyrics to a song. Trust your intuitive filters to bring you what you need or long to know. You will know you have connected by observing a subtle shift in the way your pet relates to you. During the communication, as I typically experience, the pet may appear relaxed or may look directly at you.

Please relay a story about your work.

Dr. Agnes Thomas—I received a call from a woman whose dog refused to eat or drink. He was so weak, that he would just lie on the floor all day. She wanted to know if he should be "put down." I asked the dog what was going on, and why he stopped eating and drinking. He said, "The water is no good."

When I related this to the woman, she didn't quite understand. I suggested that she open a can of broth and offer it to him. She did, and he drank all of it right away. I then asked the woman to get a gallon of bottled water and see if he would drink it. She called me back after she went to the store and gave him the water. She said he drank two gallons of bottled water.

I asked the woman what kind of water she had in her house, e.g., city water or well water. She answered well water. I recommended that she have it retested. She did, and it was positive for E. coli, a dangerous bacterium that can cause cholera. The dog said he was trying to tell her not to drink the water by abstaining from it himself.

The woman had other beverages that she could drink, pop, milk, juice, etc., without being exposed to the well water. The dog had nothing but the well water, so he was stricken first. The dog is a hero, not only to his owner, but to neighbors in the area sharing the same water.

Betsy Crouse—Years ago, I was house and horse sitting for my sister, who at the time had a yearling filly she had raised from birth. This youngster had learned to be respectful of and careful with my sister, but she had not, at that time, had lots of exposure to people in general, and her manners with humans at large were sorely lacking.

It was evening, and I had done the chores and was ready to let the three horses in through the sliding back door of the barn. I slid the door open, and there they were, hungry for their supper. As soon as the opening was wide enough, the filly stepped right into my space. She would have pushed me aside if I'd allowed it, but I squawked indignantly, throwing my arms up to block her passage. She retreated slightly, but immediately made another try. I again made it clear that she was not to mow me down, and she again retreated, though reluctantly. She made a third try, and I said, "You WILL NOT come into this barn until I say you may come!" Then I closed the door, and went back into the barn for several minutes.

Returning to the door, I opened it again, expecting a more mannerly response. Instead, the filly tried once again to run me over. At that point I said, loudly and clearly, "You will BACK UP from this door, WALK over to that fence, and WAIT until the others have come in, THEN you may come in and eat!" I repeated the same sequence three times, each time being met with pushy efforts from the filly, and each time delivering my message, now silently, but with equal strength and unwavering conviction. I don't know where my conviction came from, since my request was completely unreasonable in standard training terms. But I'd had it with being trampled and wasn't feeling all that reasonable.

My mind was focused with laser–like clarity, and on the fourth try, the filly stood her ground when I opened the door. I repeated my decree, and she backed up several steps, turned to her right, walked fifteen feet to the edge of the barn, and stood with her head over the fence. I let her grandma and then her mom past me, as I knew they'd walk right to their own stalls and go in. She then came to the door, let me take her by the halter, and walked with me to her stall, where I let her go in to her supper. You could have knocked me over with a feather.

Renee Takacs—One of my first cases was a horse who kept walking mostly toward the left. The owner called me and asked for a reading. The veterinarian couldn't find anything wrong with its legs. When I placed myself mentally inside of the horse's body, I couldn't see very well out of my right eye. When the owner relayed this to the barn veterinarian, she discovered the horse was developing a cataract! I was amazed to have helped the veterinarian discover this condition and grateful to be able to help the horse receive the proper attention. As with people, my intent is to receive information that is helpful or need-to-know in order to avoid unnecessary suffering.

Intuitive Heart Pet Connection

Henry Reed, Ph.D., is a pioneer in the area of intuition and psychic development. One clear mission in his life has been to help others tap into and channel their psychic potential. To this end he has developed a simple "Intuitive Heart" technique for connecting with and gaining intuitive information from another person. A more in-depth look at this practice can be gained from Dr. Reed's book, *The Intuitive Heart*.

With Henry Reed's permission, I have adapted his Intuitive Heart method to apply to a human–animal heart connection. The following is a guide to help you connect with and intuit impressions from your pet, but this technique may serve several purposes. Through this process you can gain helpful insights, such as the purpose of your relationship. You can also use the heart connection to channel healing energy to your pet. Also, you can use the link from time to time simply to strengthen your overall pet connection.

If you choose to use this technique to get information, start by formulating a question. It is best to have an open-ended question, asking for a lesson or insight rather than limiting the answer to something specific like yes or no. A question like, "How do you feel about the new cat I brought home?" is better than, "Do you like the new cat I brought home?" When you come up with your question, write it on a piece of paper, slip it into a pocket, and put it out of your mind.

Now, get comfortable with your pet. Sit with him on your lap, lie with him on the floor, or whatever. Let the petting and nuzzling and squirming subside. Let your friend know that you are going to spend some quiet time together. I find that having a hand on my pet's chest, feeling his heart, aids the heart connection.

Initiate an intuitive mode of functioning by closing your eyes and shifting your attention to the breath. Relax and let the breath flow naturally and unaided. With each breath, relax further. Let any preconceived thoughts fall away. An affirmation for this step might be, "I can trust in inspiration." These words are used to remind you that it is not necessary to force intuition, for it will come on its own, spontaneously and naturally.

Next, shift your attention to your heart and experience the feeling of warmth and love, gradually letting this feeling expand toward the pet's heart, creating a fantasy of two hearts joined in love. The affirmation for this step might be, "I give myself permission to care enough for this animal to share in the feeling of love and to share of myself with this pet."

Then, if you are looking to acquire information, allow a personal memory to spontaneously come to mind, trusting that it will be a memory that will prove useful to understanding your pet. The affirmation for this step would be, "I now allow to enter into my awareness a memory that will stimulate in me insights that will prove helpful to my understanding of my companion."

Now, accept the first memory that comes to mind, no matter how trivial, embarrassing, or seemingly irrelevant. The memory may appear to have absolutely nothing to do with the pet or the situation. Describe this thought to yourself, as if telling a story. After describing this event, ponder what lesson this experience has to offer. In an improvisational manner, speaking from the heart, in other words, fashion an insight from what you can now learn from that experience. When you feel finished with the session, reread the original question and see how the insight you gained corresponds to the inquiry.

If instead of getting information you wish to channel healing energy, after forming the heart connection, imagine energy flowing into your body from the Divine and passing into your pet through the conduit you have formed. You might choose the affirmation, "I am a channel of blessings for this companion." Allow yourself to feel the energy flow for as long as seems comfortable—a few seconds or several minutes. End the session with a prayer of thanks.

If neither healing nor information are sought, simply enjoy the heart connection with your pet. However, do pay attention to any thoughts, feelings, or memories that may surface spontaneously. Just because you do not seek to communicate with your pet does not mean he does not have something to say to you.

The first time I made this connection with my cat Blaze I did not have an issue to address. I simply made the connection and got the image of tongues of fire. As I thought about what this might mean I realized that he is a Flame Point Siamese named Blaze. I got the feeling he liked his image. With my dog, DJ, as soon as I began to make the heart connection, he would squirm. Interestingly, he has a heart condition. I found that I had to make the connection very gently. Once connected, I chose to channel healing energy to him.

When I linked up with Apple, our eighteen-year-old cat, I had the question, "Why are you a part of my life?" A memory came to mind of playing games while riding my bike as a child. It was a happy time when things were not as serious as they seem today. The lesson I came up with is that play and balance are important in life. I think that Apple does remind me from time to time not to take myself too seriously and to have fun once in awhile.

Tuning in to your pet's world both physically and intuitively strengthens the bond you share. Keeping in touch will help to ensure that you are clearly understood, making cohabitation more enjoyable.

As with any relationship involving shared quarters, the behavior of each party can become an issue. A pet connection is especially prone to such problems because in many ways we are so different from our companions. Sometimes the way we act speaks louder than words. Let's take our communication to the next level and explore behavior modification.

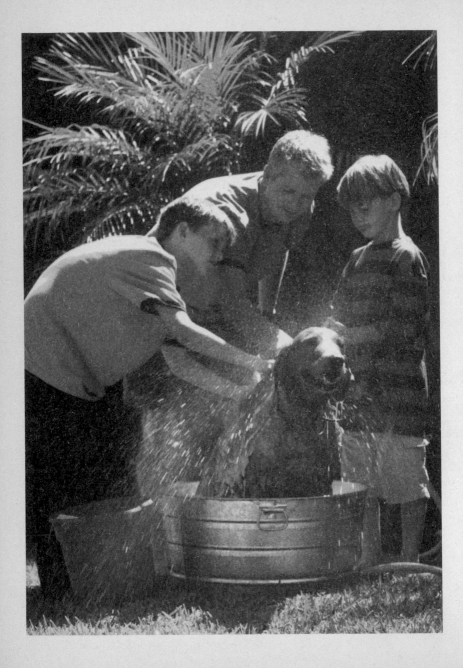

CHAPTER

4

BEHAVIOR MODIFICATION

The *training*, then, may be in accord with the tendencies and thus bring harmony, peace, and an influence worth while, or the entity may be trained in opposition to tendencies and bring consternation and troubled conditions in the entity's experience;...

759-1

Animal caregivers are often perplexed if not perturbed by the behavior of their pets. In fact, most of the millions of animals that are euthanized at animal shelters every year are killed because of behavioral problems. This statistic testifies to a very important, potential breakdown in the pet connection. Certainly something must be done to stop the slaughter.

When we talk about behavior modification we are speaking of training. However, the word training has a very one-sided connotation. We train animals, subjugating them to our wills. The term behavior modification is intentionally ambiguous. Whose behavior are we going to change—ours or that of our pets'?

In general the animals that we care for want to please us. The problem is that we often send such mixed messages that they do not understand what we want from them. For example, many people find it cute to have their little puppy jump up on them as a greeting when they come home from work. This behavior is rewarded and reinforced by the caregiver who lavishes praise and love on the exuberant pup.

Unfortunately, when the little fur ball grows into a 150–pound German shepherd, suddenly this same behavior that had previously been encouraged is considered obnoxious and even dangerous. The dog gets blamed and punished for the problem when the responsibility clearly rests on the owner.

We need to change our behavior in order to modify our pets' behavior. This process is really an extension of animal communication. We are simply communicating in special ways in order to achieve specific results.

Holistic training is a process that involves all of yourself and your pet. You must communicate mentally as well as verbally and physically. Keep a clear picture in your mind of the behavior you want to see. Be sure your body language, verbal commands, and mental pictures are consistent.

Holistic training also means instruction that honors our animal companions for who they are. Each species has its tendencies. Each breed has certain characteristics. Every individual has his own unique personality. All of these factors must be considered when dealing with behavior issues.

Animals are sentient beings. In the wild, they are required to hunt in order to eat. Hunting is both physically and mentally challenging. Our pets, on the other hand, are often left alone for long periods and have their food handed to them. Where is the challenge in that?

It should not be a surprise that bored and lonely animals find mischievous ways of occupying their time. Many behavior problems can be prevented or solved simply by giving the pet more attention and by offering physical and mental challenges such as those involved with training and playing. A tired, contented animal is not likely to seek out destructive ways to vent his energy.

There are certain behaviors that we are not likely to train out of our pets. We cannot expect a cat not to scratch. We can, however, train him to use a scratching post instead of our furniture. Dogs are naturally going to chew on something. We can't stop the chewing; however, we can teach them what is acceptable to chew on and what is not.

Because each pet connection is unique, one technique does not fit all. You must determine what works best in your situation. Which techniques best match your personal style and your pet's personality. If one training course is not working, try another course with a different instructor and a different approach.

As we look at training from a holistic perspective, the process becomes one of education. We educate ourselves about our pets and their unique needs. At the same time we educate our animal friends about what is expected of them in order to live happily together.

Unless educated otherwise, dogs and cats will behave according to their natures. A dog does not automatically know that it is supposed to defecate only outside. A cat does not naturally scratch only on scratching posts. It is not fair to expect animals to live by our rules if we do not teach them the rules.

The goal of behavior modification is to conduct ourselves in such a way that our pets can express who they are but do it in a way that we can live with. Before exploring specific training concepts, let's investigate the instinctive behaviors of dogs and cats.

Normal Animal Behavior

Most of what we consider to be animal behavioral problems are really normal animal conduct. We need to understand our pets' behavior from their point of view and not judge what they do based on our

standards. The cat that urinates on the clean laundry is not being venge-
ful. The dog that nips the grandson did not do it out of jealousy. Animals have their own priorities and their ways are rarely due to
humanlike motives. To understand, train, and live happily with our
animal companions we need to realize what makes them tick.

A major motivating force in cats is their territorial nature. This is a
tendency that we should be able to relate to. We lock our doors, put
fences up, and even etch our social security numbers into our personal
property to claim it as ours. We are made uneasy by strangers who
invade our private space. Cats feel the same way.

The feline, scent-based territorial tendency is deeply entrenched and
begins at birth. When kittens nurse, each one claims her own nipple.
Every time the kittens go to feed, even without the ability to see or hear,
they are guided back to their personal food supply by their sense of
smell. If the kittens are removed and the mother's belly is cleaned thoroughly, removing all the scent, the kittens return confused and may
even struggle over the same nipple. From birth cats use scent to claim
their territory and feel comfortable in their environment.

The problem for us comes in the way our cats express their need for
private property. One way is through urine marking and another is
through scratching. When the target of these destructive behaviors is
our furniture, walls, carpeting, and drapes, problems begin. Yet, cats
need to scratch; they need to urinate; and they need to feel secure in
their surroundings. Can we reach a compromise?

It is also part of a cat's nature to be nocturnal. A normal cat rests all
day long and becomes active at night. Unfortunately, this schedule does
not usually mesh well with our own. Many of us find it highly irritating
to be disturbed in the middle of the night by our kitty friends playing
ninja warrior on our beds. Do we really have to put up with this?

Finally, felines are active hunters. Their predatory instinct cannot be
denied. If your cat cannot find birds or rodents to stalk and attack, your
feet will do just fine. How do we deal with such insolence? We will
discuss solutions to these feline behavior disputes later in this chapter.

Our canine friends confront us with a whole other set of challenges.
Dogs are ruled by their pack nature. Again, this is a tendency that we

are all familiar with. (It is a dog–eat–dog world after all.) Each dog seeks to claim his position in the hierarchy. Most everything the dog does, from mounting behavior to rushing out the front door ahead of you, is a statement of dominance. Remember, the top dog does not have to take orders from anyone. So how do we command the respect of our dogs and remain best friends?

Each breed of dog has different characteristic behaviors that they have been bred for. Some dig for a living, while some herd other animals. Some are aggressive and others just bark a lot. It is also normal for all dogs, especially puppies, to chew on things. What do we do about some of these obnoxious canine behaviors?

Fundamental Educational Guidelines

Animals do not readily understand human language. Even in the hands of an expert animal communicator, dogs and cats learn best by experience. Even though the pet may know what you want from him, he may need to be motivated to comply. A behavior that results in an immediate, unpleasant penalty will be avoided in the future. A behavior that results in immediate, pleasant consequences will be repeated and soon becomes a habit. By its very nature a habit gets reiterated automatically, without thinking about it.

Although animals do not comprehend our speech, they do pick up on our thoughts, feelings, and emotions. It is imperative to maintain a positive attitude while training your pet. Your companion can and will learn the lesson. It is also helpful to visualize the desired behavior instead of concentrating on what you do not want to happen. Filling your mind with past disappointments will only serve to hinder the training process.

Animals can reason to a limited extent but do not project thought into the future or into the past. They consistently live in the present. They have no concept of the long–term consequences of their deeds. A cat does not think, "Gee, I had better not scratch the couch because when my caregiver gets home she'll be angry." They also do not project their thought back in time. If you rub your puppy's nose in the feces it deposited on the living room carpet while you were at work, he does not understand that his having pooped in the house resulted in this unpleasant outcome. The only thing you teach the pup by this act is that sometimes when you come home you are nasty and irrational.

The easiest way to educate our pets is through immediate rewards for good behavior and negative consequences for bad behavior. Practically speaking, rewarding appropriate behavior works much better than punishing misdeeds. Positive reinforcement is how experts train wild animals. Can you imagine what would happen if dolphins were trained by smacking them on the nose every time they didn't jump through the hoop? "Bad, bad dolphin!" I don't think they would ever catch on.

There are many reasons to avoid punishing pets. Our forms and means of punishment are often misunderstood by our pets. Pets do not understand screaming. Their mothers never yelled at them. Animals have more subtle and more effective ways of expressing displeasure. Yelling at pets usually just excites and confuses them causing them to behave even more irrationally.

Often when we think we are punishing a pet, we are actually rewarding their bad behavior.

Cleo is a young, spry kitty with an abundance of energy. She has gotten into the habit of sneaking up on her owner, Bob, at 3:00 a.m. while he is sleeping. Cleo jumps on his feet through the covers and attacks as a good nocturnal predator should. Understandably, the startled Bob jumps out of bed to wrestle Cleo into submission. He thinks he has punished the cat, but Cleo has gotten just what she was looking for; a little action on an otherwise boring night. You can bet Cleo will be up to the challenge again.

The timing of the punishment is especially important. Remember that animals are affected by the immediate consequences of their deeds. If you hear your cat scratching the couch and rush in and scare her, but you arrive just as she is stopping, she may think she is being punished for quitting. She'll have to do a better job next time.

A second problem with the above example is that in such cases the cat quickly associates the punishment with you. At best your cat learns, "I guess I shouldn't ever scratch the furniture—when she's around." You have succeeded in teaching your cat not to destroy your house in your presence. This lesson works only if you never leave the cat unattended.

A final problem with punishment in general is that it is not very specific. There are hundreds of wrong behaviors. Punishing the cat for scratching the couch leaves it wide open to scratch the love seat, recliner, walls, drapes, etc. On the other hand there is only one right behavior—scratching the scratching post. It makes much more sense to reward the one right behavior rather than punish the numerous incorrect behaviors.

As for corporal punishment; this practice is doomed to fail. Hitting or otherwise harming an animal to correct her only adds aggression and violence to the equation. When you multiply this by the upset emotional state of the trainer who employs such means, you have a recipe for disaster. The Edgar Cayce readings agree with eliminating corporal punishment.

> As we find, punishment of a corporal nature is often bad; more often harmful than helpful. The activities, then, should be not so much as "Don't" but "Do" ... for kindness goes much farther than stress. Positive kindness.   758-27

The bottom line is that direct punishment of any sort does not work well in training animals. We will, however, discuss some ways of indirectly discouraging your pet from doing unwanted behaviors.

So the best way to communicate what we would like our pets to do is through rewarding the desired behavior. Do your best to catch your pet doing something right. Your animal communication skills will help guide your pet while the reward reinforces the behavior until it becomes a habit.

There are a few principles about rewards that need to be understood to increase their effectiveness. First of all, rewards should be given periodically and not after each and every correct response. Rewards need to be given frequently when a lesson is first being taught, but less frequently as the animal learns. The concept of periodic rewards is what keeps casinos in business. If you got a coin out every time you put a coin into the slot machine, the game would become boring after awhile. It is that periodic reward that keeps the gambler coming back even though he is losing more than he gained.

Another principle of rewards is that the type of compensation needs to change frequently. Food rewards work well, but praise, petting, play, and other desirable activities are just as rewarding. Again, the education process is more fun when it involves a variety of activities and treats as rewards.

Yet another training guideline is that prevention is the key. The earlier you can help your pet establish good habits the better. It is much easier to train a puppy or kitten to do the right thing than it is to untrain an adult animal from doing the wrong thing. Basic training starts from day one and continues for the life of the pet.

Never take a good habit for granted. Without reinforcement, animals will sometimes revert back to their natural tendencies. This does not mean you have to pop a treat to your pet every time it does the right thing. Still, it is a good idea to reward good behaviors periodically throughout the life of the animal.

One more helpful concept for animal education is the appropriate use of confinement. Confinement is not imprisonment and is not a form of punishment. It serves several useful purposes. Confinement protects pets from injuring or poisoning themselves. At the same time, it protects your property from destructive behavior. Confinement helps break a pet's bad habits by denying access to the inciting stimuli. Finally, it promotes the formation of good habits by directing the pet's behavior to proper channels.

Confinement takes different forms for cats versus dogs. Cats are kept in a single room with food, water, litter box, bed, toys, and scratching posts. Dogs are confined in kennels or crates. This small area for canines capitalizes on their natural denning instinct. The proper use of confinement will be discussed later in this chapter.

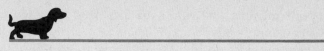

Starting Off on the Right Paw

When starting out with a new pet, it is essential to set the ground rules from the beginning. An ounce of prevention is worth a pound of cure. This old saying is especially true when beginning a pet connection with a young animal. How a pet is treated during its first few months of age affects his behavior for life. Before getting into the training aspects of beginning with your new companion, we'll examine other initial considerations for cats and dogs.

An important primary idea is that of getting the pet on a set feeding schedule. Leaving food out for pets to graze on is not a good idea. It is much better to get your pet used to eating at set times from the start.

Establishing meal times helps to eliminate begging. I have cat patients who nag their caregivers whenever their food bowls are empty. The cats cry demandingly until the beleaguered person complies. Of course, by giving in, the hapless human reinforces this obnoxious behavior. The feline learns that harassment works. Animals that are fed on a schedule realize that begging is futile. The food is only given at meal times.

Another advantage of set feeding times is that you have more control over how much food your pet is eating. This way obesity can be avoided. Multiple pets can be fed at the same time but in different rooms eliminating the problem of one eating the other's food. You also have more accurate information about your pet's appetite. You know right away whether or not she is eating.

Dogs who are fed free choice seem to take their food for granted. They appreciate and respect you much more when they know you are the giver of food. It is also easier to housetrain a puppy who is fed on schedule. Dogs have to urinate and defecate about twenty to thirty minutes after eating. If you know when your dog eats, you know when to take him out. Thus you set him up for success in the housetraining department.

To start off, remember that young animals need to be fed three to four times a day. Simply put the food down and take it up after twenty minutes. If your pet does not eat, she will have to wait until the next meal time. Soon she will catch on and eat as soon as the food is served. In fact, she will remind you when it is dinner time.

Kitty Care

At the beginning of a pet connection with a cat it is essential to realize their territorial nature. Whether adult or kitten, a new cat can become overwhelmed by a large new territory. The new kitty should be kept in one room at first. This should be considered a play room similar to a child's play pen. Everything your new friend needs is right there as mentioned above. Also be sure to provide hiding places such as boxes in case she is shy. It is wise to confine a feline for the first few weeks in a new house. Keeping kitty in one room of the house helps to get off on the right foot in a number of ways.

First of all, the kitty will be in close proximity to the litter boxes so it is more likely to use them. It will certainly have fewer wrong places to urinate. Because the captive feline does not have access to your couch and other furniture, it cannot get used to scratching them. Instead, she has only fun scratching posts to use; so, with your encouragement, she will get into good habits.

If you already have other cats, the play room is especially important. It not only allows the new kitty to get used to a small territory first, it also allows your current pets time to get used to the smell of a new cat before actually confronting her. During the confinement be sure to spend extra time with your pre-existing cats to reassure them that they are still loved and everything is going to be all right.

Once the new kitty feels safe and secure in her play room, gradually open up more and more of the house for her to explore. If you have current cat residents, be sure that the initial encounters are controlled. Have someone holding each cat and just let them see and smell each other the first few times. Once the time seems right, allow them to interact. Expect some hissing and spitting in the beginning. At this point it is best to let them work out their differences without interfering. Third party mediation will only extend the time it takes for the two to become buddies.

Canine Considerations

When handling a new dog, you must keep in mind their unique nature. Wild dogs live in confined dens. Crate training capitalizes on a dog's natural denning instinct. A den is a safe environment that becomes home for the dog. A crate re-creates this secure space, plus keeps the pup safe from hazards of the home and the home safe from destructive behaviors.

Dogs appreciate the controlled, structured environment the crate provides. Often, as the puppy grows and freedom is earned, the dog will return on his own to the crate for a nap or to escape from the kids.

Crate training can greatly ease housebreaking. Left on his own, a puppy will poop and pee whenever and wherever it is convenient—for him. However, puppies learn from their mothers not to eliminate where they sleep. Crating teaches the puppy to hold rather than eliminate.

Crating also allows a puppy some quiet time. When the puppy gets too rambunctious, crating him will help him settle down. Nevertheless, the crate should never be used for punishment.

The first key to crate training is to get the right crate. Find one that is airline approved. The crate should be just large enough for the puppy to stand in, turn around and lie flat on his side. If you decide to get a crate that your dog can use when he grows up, you'll need to block off the back half to make it smaller while he's a pup. Otherwise, the large size will allow him to lie at one end and eliminate at the other.

Next, place the crate in a room of the house where the dog can see most of what's going on. Do not put paper in the crate, just a few favorite toys. Also, do not put water in a puppy's crate fo help avoid accidents.

Puppies can begin training at eight weeks of age. Introduce the pup and put him in while telling him, "Kennel up." He will probably whine a little, but will soon settle down. Do not talk to or acknowledge the puppy while crated, as this will just make him anxious. After a few minutes, let him out. Be sure not to let him out while he is whining or you will be reinforcing the wrong behavior.

At first, keep the crate times short. This lets the puppy know that the confinement is not permanent. Gradually increase the amount of time he is crated, keeping in mind that young puppies need to eliminate frequently. If a young dog is left in a crate all day while you are at work, he will have no choice but to eliminate where he sleeps, even though it goes against his nature. If this continues to happen, the puppy will get used to sleeping in a soiled bed and the purpose of the crate will be defeated.

By four to six months of age your puppy can be left in the crate for up to five or six hours. Soon, as the comfortable time grows, your pup will be happy to kennel up, especially if you give him a small treat each time he complies.

The puppy should be crated whenever you are unable to watch him, when you go to bed and when you leave the house. He should only be crated for a few hours at a time during the day, and his collar should be removed for safety. Don't forget to exercise your pup before and after crating. The security of a crate does not replace the puppy's need for being part of the family. Let him participate, enjoy, and share.

Another canine tendency that I have mentioned is that dogs are pack animals. In a pack, it is important to establish a hierarchy. The top dog rules. Many people become subordinate to their dogs and do not even know it. These unruly pets soon do not obey and cannot be handled. And it all started when they were cute little puppies.

Dogs have many ways of establishing their pecking order. Often, very important messages are sent simply by the tone of voice. When a mother dog corrects her pups, she does it with a growl. A man's voice is naturally deep and mimics the mother's corrective growl. Women and children's voices are high pitched and sound more like the whining of littermates. Littermates can be dominated. This is why many puppies do not listen to the women and children in the family.

Your puppy needs to understand his place in his new pack. He must see the family members as being dominant. We do not want to create a puppy that cowers in fear when he sees you, but he must obey you. Remember, if you are not dominant, you are subordinate. No one listens to the inferior animal.

One way that one dog establishes dominance over another is by holding the muzzle of the subordinate in his mouth. Try this easy dominance exercise with your pup when he is unruly. Use your thumb and forefinger to gently encircle his muzzle. (Be sure he can breathe.) Put your face right up to his and look him right in the eyes. Tell him "settle down" in a low, deep, drawn out voice.

It is likely that the pup will cry and carry on for a few seconds. If you let go at this point then you have just taught him that if he throws a tantrum he will get his way. You must gently hold on until he settles down. As soon as he is still, let go and praise him. It is important to do this exercise with love and not out of anger. Dogs can sense your emotions and you will have a loving companion only if you treat him lovingly.

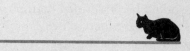

Basic Training

Initial education must be directed at three basic areas. Temperament training helps the pet deal with the various social situations that may arise. Behavior training governs laying the ground rules for acceptable behavior in general. Obedience training teaches the animal to respond to specific commands. Let's take a look at each of these and how they apply to dogs and cats.

Temperament Training

An animal's temperament refers to how it responds in various social situations. The dog that always bites kids and the cat that will not allow anyone to pet it are both exhibiting temperament problems. Although each animal comes into the world with certain temperamental tendencies, the bulk of a pet's social behavior is determined by how it is handled while very young. An animal's social behavior patterns are set by four to five months of age. It is very difficult to change a pet's temperament after this time.

This does not mean that every shy or fearful pet must have been abused and tortured as a youngster. Socially aberrant animals may have been born that way or they may simply have not been properly temperament trained at an early age.

Temperament training involves getting the young animal used to situations it is likely to find itself in later in life. Every puppy and kitten should interact with strangers (both male and female), children and other animals. These encounters need to be arranged under controlled circumstances so that the young pet is not traumatized by an exuberant child or rambunctious dog.

Young animals should be gently handled by the owner and strangers. Toes should be lightly squeezed, mouths opened, ears examined, tails tugged on—in short, anything you may need to do to an adult animal should be performed on the youngster.

Trips to the veterinary office can be made more pleasant for the life of the pet by handling the first few properly. First of all, be sure your pet is hungry. Then bring plenty of her favorite treats. All the time the pet is in the waiting room, while in the exam room, even while getting any shots, give treats generously. Soon the pet will look forward to these visits and the treats can be tapered off.

Get your kitten used to being put in a carrier. Get both puppies and kitties used to riding in the car. Be sure to drive them someplace pleasant periodically. If the only time a pet goes into a carrier or goes in the car is to be taken to the veterinarian, you can be sure they will learn to associate these experiences with the doctor's office. Then any uncertainty they may feel begins before they even get to the vets.

It is important that temperament training sessions be seen as pleasant experiences by the animal. The exercises should be accompanied by lots of love, petting, and food treats. The pet needs to be eased into the experience; so the caregiver must progress slowly and not force any pet into an uncomfortable situation. Multiple, short lessons are more effective than long, overwhelming sessions.

Another temperament issue that is a growing problem in adult dogs is a mental aberration called separation anxiety. When left alone, some dogs go berserk, chewing furniture and soiling the house. These poor pets seem to have an uncontrollable need to be with someone at all times.

It is possible that this obsession begins with how the dog was treated as a puppy. Puppies who are smothered with attention and do not learn to play independently are likely to have problems as adults. Obedience or performance training will also probably help. Animals need a sense of purpose. They need to have something else to live for besides their owners. I think all dogs naturally desire not just to be good, but good for something.

Behavior Training

Our pets' general behavior is the most important issue we deal with on a daily basis. Instinctive animal activities must be tempered to fit life with a human family. At the same time, we must realize their needs for certain behaviors and meet them half way.

For example, some dogs dig. In fact, all terriers have been bred to dig. You cannot expect that such a dog can be trained not to dig. At the same time, you should not be expected to tolerate huge holes throughout your yard and garden. What is the middle ground in this dispute?

Why not just start out by making a sand box in an out-of-the-way area of your yard for Digger to use? To entice Digger to use it, bury treats and bones in the sand. The dog will think he's found a gold mine. With repeated success at digging in the sand he will see no point in digging anywhere else.

Dog Behavior Training—There are some special behavior issues concerning dogs. Dogs especially must be desensitized about their food bowls. Sometimes dogs become food aggressive and may lash out at anyone who approaches their full food container. This is an especially dangerous situation when children are involved. To prevent this problem, get the puppy used to having people around his bowl while he is eating. Even go as far as placing his food into his bowl one handful at a time. This way the canine learns that it is good to have hands near the food bowl because that is where the food comes from.

House training is another uniquely canine necessity. For this task, the first thing you need to realize is that puppies do not instinctively know that they are supposed to relieve themselves outside. The dining room carpet looks like a fine place to them, or anywhere else they get the urge. You need to give them a reason to do it in the right place. This is where positive reinforcement comes in.

Next, you need to think like a dog. Let me explain. The most common mistake people make when house training is that they take the dog out for a walk to relieve himself. Now, become the dog. You are walking around and playing outside just the way you like to. Then you squat to do your business and the next thing you know you are getting dragged back into the house.

Well, it does not take the dog equivalent of a rocket scientist to figure out that the longer you hold it, the more fun you get to have outside. Before you know it, you can hold it for a long time while outside having fun. Finally the owner thinks you must not have to do anything so he takes you back in the house. That is when you realize that your bladder is full and, uh oh! There goes the dining room carpet.

To housebreak a puppy effectively you need to take the dog out on a leash every time he goes out. You need to go to the same spot in the yard each time so the puppy associates that spot with potty time. It even helps to have a one word command, such as "potty," to further cue the puppy. (Be sure to choose a word that you do not use in casual conversation.)

Now just stand there with the puppy on the leash. No playing, no walking, no anything. Eventually the puppy will relieve himself. Then, throw a party, give him praise, give him a treat, take him for a walk, let him know he did the right thing. Soon, the puppy will potty outside ASAP to get the reward.

Do not make the mistake of sending the puppy outside to do his business and then giving him a treat when he comes back in. Because the reward was not given immediately after the desired behavior, the puppy will not associate the treat with the act of eliminating. The puppy only learns that going out and in means treat time, so he will soon pester you to let him out and in frequently, with or without eliminating.

Here are some other pointers. Never punish the dog by rubbing his nose in his mistakes. All the animal learns from this is that when you find poop on the floor, you turn into a cruel person. They cannot reason out their part in the incident. Correction is only helpful if you catch the dog in "the act." At that time you should yell, "Outside!" The shock of this will tighten every sphincter in the animal's body plus convey the right place to go. Then take the animal out and proceed as indicated above.

Furthermore, vary the rewards to keep the process interesting for the pup. Keep the puppy with you or in a crate when in the house to deter any mistakes. Take the puppy out at least every hour, since young animals do not have the control needed to hold their waste in for long periods. (This tip is very important but can be impossible for those who work, a fact that needs to be considered when timing the arrival of a new puppy.) If the pet does not potty within five minutes of being outside, take him directly inside and try later.

Finally, as mentioned earlier, feeding the puppy at set times helps. Most puppies have to relieve themselves twenty to thirty minutes after eating; so a feeding schedule allows you to synchronize the potty time with the puppy's natural urges.

Remember to be patient. Some puppies, just like some children, are more difficult to potty train than others. A little time spent on training now will pay off as a lifetime of pleasant behavior.

Biting is another puppy behavior that needs to be modified. Puppies bite. It is just something they do. They bite furniture, shoes, and hands. Just like children, they seem to want to put everything into their mouths. So, there are two issues; biting objects and biting people.

To discourage your puppy from biting objects, be sure to provide him with chew toys. Again, it is better to train the puppy to chew the right thing that to keep punishing him for chewing the wrong thing. More is not necessarily better when it comes to toys. It is better to keep the toys new and interesting.

The best way to utilize a number of chew toys is to rotate them in and out of use. Always keep some toys hidden and every week, bring those out and hide the others. For the puppy it is like having something new every week. The use of hollow chew toys into which treats can be stuffed is also helpful. Puppies and even adult dogs can be occupied for hours trying to get the treats out.

If you do not want personal items such as your shoes to be destroyed, do not give your puppy an old sneaker to chew on. Your puppy cannot distinguish between your old gym shoe and your new Nike's. If you allow him to chew on one you are inviting him to chew on the other.

As far as biting people, again this is an expected activity, but one that needs to be shaped. If puppies are playing together and one bites the other too hard, the wounded pup yips sharply and scampers away. The offender is left alone. The game is over. Soon he learns that rough play ends the fun.

You can use a similar tactic when your puppy is playing with and biting you. Every time he bites hard say, "Ouch" and leave the room. As the puppy catches on, he will bite with less force. Gradually reduce the amount of pressure you tolerate until the puppy is simply mouthing you. Now your pup will learn the type of biting that is acceptable for humans.

Cat Behavior Training—Train your kitty to be an indoor cat. Cats are much better off when kept strictly inside the house. It is a dangerous world out there. Kitties that are allowed outdoors are susceptible to injuries from other animals and cars, life–threatening infections such as Feline Leukemia Virus, and poisoning from antifreeze and other toxins. Outdoor cats also may cause property damage or they might bring fleas into the house. Although it seems only natural for a cat to be outside climbing trees and chasing birds, she will live longer if kept inside.

While living indoors, cats need to have certain natural behaviors tamed just as dogs do. If left to her own devices, a cat can destroy a house with scratching and house soiling. As previously mentioned, it is much easier to prevent such behavior rather than to eradicate a bad habit.

While the new cat is in confinement, be sure to reinforce her use of the scratching post and litter box. Play with the kitty only around her scratching post so she learns to like being around it. Drag her favorite toys up and down the post to encourage her to dig into it. Never force a cat to scratch. Making the training session a play session is much more effective.

Spend as much time as you can in the play room with your cat. This will allow you to determine her litter box schedule. Set feedings will also help with the timing. Every time you catch her using her box, praise her and give her a treat. Do not take any good behavior for granted.

As predators, cats have a lot of pent–up energy. Is it any wonder that cats sometimes stalk and attack their caregivers? Occasionally, a cute little kitty can assault with such ferocity that they injure their human friend. Every cat has this predator tendency although they all express it to different degrees. Wild felines spend the majority of their time hunting. Because their captive counterparts do not need to hunt to eat, we need to find other ways to fulfill their innate desire to hunt and thwart an aggressive tendency.

The solution is as fun as it is effective. Play with the kitty. Drag and dangle toys to mimic prey and let the kitten go at it. Ample play sessions are required for cats of all ages but especially young kittens. Another way to help avoid the development of an aggressive cat is to bring home two kittens. That way the kitties play with each other and are much less likely to molest their caregiver.

The nocturnal nature of cats can lead to frustration if not nipped in the bud. Again the solution is play. Keep the cat awake and active during the day. Have an especially long play session just before bedtime to tire her out. A played–out, content kitty is not apt to be destructive or nocturnally energetic. It is funny how play is the solution to so many problems.

Obedience Training

The concept of teaching a pet how to respond to specific commands applies mostly to dogs. Sure, it might be fun to have a cat that sits and heels when directed to, but what's the point? For dogs this training is essential.

Training puppies to obey should begin as soon as they are weaned. Many dog–training clubs have puppy classes that can be very beneficial.

Puppy training classes are mostly geared toward socialization of the puppy. In other words, they help the puppy feel comfortable around strange dogs and strange people. Some puppy classes also help with obedience training. The sooner your puppy learns to listen to you, the better off you will both be. Whether or not you enroll in a class, a few hours a week working with your puppy will pay off as a lifetime of good behavior.

The simplest way to start with your puppy is to teach him to sit. Make him sit for everything (before he gets to go outside, before he gets his food, before he gets petted, etc.). Soon the puppy learns that sitting is a way of asking for something. This technique is invaluable for several reasons.

Teaching a dog to sit before any positive experience helps to establish your dominance. Such training lets him know that he must comply to get what he wants. Also, a dog that sits to get petted will sit as a greeting instead of jumping on you. He can't sit and jump on you at the same time, so by reinforcing the sit you can deter obnoxious behavior.

In order to teach a puppy to sit, use a treat as a lure. Hold the treat right in front of his nose and slowly raise your hand up and back over the top of his head while saying, "Sit." As his nose goes up, his rear will naturally go down. Visualize the desired posture. When he sits, praise him and give him the treat. Never force a dog's rear end down by pushing on it. Furthermore, only give the command once. Otherwise your puppy will learn that "sit sit sit sit" means "sit" and will not obey until you spit out the fourth "sit."

Once he has the sit command down, you can teach him to stay. To do this, start with him in a sit position. Tell him to stay and move back just a foot or two and only for a few seconds. Again, hold a picture in your mind of the puppy remaining seated. Then move back and give praise and rewards. Gradually up the ante by moving farther and having him hold the stay longer. Be sure to keep the training sessions fun.

Now with the sit and stay under his belt it is time to move on to "come." For this it is necessary to have a long lead on the puppy. The lead enforces the command. Some puppies think it is more fun to play chase than to come when called. If you tell your puppy to come and he runs the other way and you chase him, you have just taught him that "come" means let's play chase.

Of course, if your puppy is hungry and having fun and you have treats, he is not likely to run the other way. But, sometimes mischief gets the better of a pup, so keep a leash on him. Now, put him in a sit–stay and move a very short distance. Then say "come" and call his name. Crouch down, clap your hands, and make him want to come. If he does not, gently pull him with the leash. Gradually increase the distance.

In addition, periodically ask your puppy to come during play. Be sure you have the other end of the leash. The idea is to be sure he will come no matter what he is up to. Of course, food treats and lots of praise will encourage compliance. Soon your puppy will pay attention and obey your every command.

The above obedience commands are important for every dog to ad-here to. When a dog sits and stays on command, many bad behaviors such as jumping up can be controlled. Any dog that is outside off leash must come when called to avoid accidents and keep him from running off.

You may wish to enroll in a canine training course. There you and your companion may learn more commands. Avoid any training that involves a lot of leash jerking and other heavy–handed measures. Most training can be done with positive reinforcement.

One particular positive training technique that is becoming popular is called clicker training. With this technique, a clicking device is used by the trainer to let the dog know exactly when he has done the right thing. Then the reward is given. The clicker allows for more precise communication and shaping of the pet's behavior.

Cats Behaving Badly

We have discussed many training and behavior issues in this chapter. Most of the common canine behavior problems have been adequately addressed in the training sections. There are a couple of feline behavior issues that need to be tackled in case it is too late to prevent the problems and the unacceptable situation needs to be remedied.

Urinary problems in cats are very common. In fact, nonuse of the litter box is the number one reason cats are left at shelters. When a cat does not use her litter box, both the caregiver and the cat have a problem.

There are several reasons that a cat may urinate outside the litter box. The first consideration is that there may be a medical problem. Cats are prone to developing crystals in their urine which can make urination painful. Urinary tract infections are also common in the feline. Both of these conditions can cause the cat to have a sudden urge to void, and if a litter box is not handy—oops.

Sugar diabetes is somewhat common in middle-aged to older cats. This disease causes the animal to drink more and urinate more. Sometimes there is such a high volume of urine that the cat can't make it to the box in time.

Other less common medical problems that can cause such accidents are the formation of bladder stones or the development of a bladder tumor. Analysis of the cat's urine and sometimes blood work and x-rays are needed to diagnose these medical conditions.

Once these diseases have been ruled out we need to consider feline behavior as the cause. As discussed previously, cats use urine to mark their territory. This is normal cat behavior. We may regard this method as madness, but I'm sure that if we asked our cats, they would have the same feeling about our use of fences.

Territorial urine marking tends to be more likely when more than one cat inhabits a single household. Having several cats in such confined quarters is not a normal situation. The fact that most cats in such a circumstance do not urine mark is amazing. A single cat might also urine mark if she is troubled by cats she sees outside. The tip off of this situation is finding puddles near windows or doors.

Unneutered male cats are most likely to urine mark, but neutered males and even spayed and unspayed females may do so as well. If your cat is unaltered, it is advisable to have her fixed. Often this procedure alone will stop the problem.

Cats also use their urine to let their caregivers know that they are upset and any change in the animal's routine may disturb her. Changes in the furniture, the carpet or even a change in the caregiver's schedule can cause much kitty consternation. Your cat might also freak out due to the arrival of house guests, invading her space.

If your cat has ever had a bad experience while in the box, she may never go back. It only takes one unpleasant event. For example, if her litter box is in the laundry room and the washer rumbles while she is in the box, her litter box training may be down the tubes. Just jumping into a messy litter box could ruin it for her. Of course, rushing to the conclusion that she is getting revenge assumes that your cat finds urine as repulsive as we do. This simply is not the case.

Do what you can to figure out what changed at the time your cat started to misbehave, and remedy the situation. The least you can do is to give her more attention. One–on–one time playing, petting, and cuddling goes a long way toward relieving cat anxiety.

Many times, even when the inciting cause of the problem has been addressed, the cat may continue to go outside the litter box out of habit. Now we need to persuade the kitty to use the litter box once again.

If your cat has chosen just a couple of choice locations to void, you can discourage the pattern by placing a piece of carpet runner—spiked side up—at the target sites. If she has multiple potty areas, then confinement is a better strategy. Lock your cat into her play room for about a month.

Be sure to keep her litter box spotlessly clean. In fact, have two litter boxes available with two different types of litter to see which one she prefers. *Hint:* Most cats like the scoopable type of litter better than plain clay. Also, nearly all cats favor unscented to scented varieties. When you find kitty's favorite litter, use only that one.

While your cat is being confined, be sure to clean and deodorize any and all potty spots in the house. I think the enzymatic cleaners work best. Ask your veterinarian for his recommendation.

Once the cat is using the litter box consistently, open up another room of the house for a few weeks. Gradually open up more and more of the house until she has free range once again. Be sure to provide one litter box per cat plus one. If you have one cat you need two litter boxes. Four cats need five boxes. Also, clean all litter boxes daily. No one likes to use a filthy toilet! And be sure the litter boxes are located in a non-threatening area of the house.

Inappropriate urination is one of the most difficult behavior problems to correct in cats. With patience, understanding and these few techniques, soon you'll have your cat once again thinking inside the box.

Scratching furniture is another big problem for cat owners. Cats need to scratch things to sharpen their claws and to stretch their muscles and tendons. They are also driven to do this as another way to mark their territory. You cannot expect a cat not to scratch things but you can teach the cat to scratch the appropriate objects.

So, the first thing to do is to have several scratching posts available for your cat. Now, just because the label says "Scratching Post" doesn't mean your cat is going to know what to do with it. To train a cat to use a scratching post, the behavior must be shaped, as mentioned previously. First reward her just for being near the post. Use a special food treat like a piece of tuna or salmon. Also, reward her with attention and affection. Gradually, she will gravitate to the post. Next, play with a toy up and down the post. As her claws dig in to catch it, reward her. Soon she will get the idea.

At the same time you are encouraging her to use the scratching post you must deter her from scratching the furniture. If there are just one or two areas she is scratching, you can place scratching posts directly in front of the target to block her from getting to it. When marking territory, cats tend to go back to the same location repeatedly. If the scratching post is there, she may begin to use it. Then very slowly—about an inch per day—the scratching post can be moved to a more convenient location.

If there are multiple scratching areas or if the above strategy does not work, there are other ways to deter the cat. Placing double sided tape or aluminum foil on the scratched areas tends to repel cats from scratching. Also, the area can be booby trapped. Put a few pennies into two soft drink cans. Tie a few strings between the cans and let the strings hang down over the scratched area. Now when the cat scratches, the cans will fall and startle her. This commotion may be enough to keep her away and break the habit. Of course, it is essential that the cat be learning the right place to scratch at the same time.

If all else fails to break her habit of scratching the furniture, confinement may be needed. Keep her in her playroom with her food, water, litter box, scratching posts, and toys. This is not meant as punishment but as a way of keeping her from her bad routine and to keep her focused on your scratching post training.

In order for mankind and beasts to live together and get along, we must address these issues of behavior—both ours and theirs. Behavior modification is the way to bring out the very best in our animal companions. As we accentuate the positive and eliminate the negative, we create a healthy, holistic relationship.

A healthy pet connection also requires physical health for our animal friends. The Edgar Cayce readings abundantly addressed the subject of holistic health for humans. Next we will explore how these concepts apply to our animals.

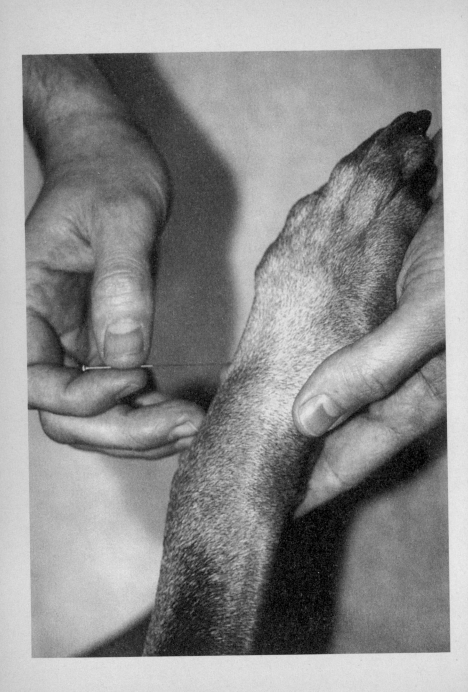

CHAPTER 5

HOLISTIC PET HEALTH

Now as we find, in considering the particular disturbances which exist with this body . . . the body *whole*
must be taken into consideration; that is, the physical,
the mental, and the spiritual attributes of the body.

1189-2

Edgar Cayce is considered by some to be the father of holistic
medicine in the United States. One reason for this is that the
majority of founding members of the American Holistic Medical Association were proponents of the Cayce health philosophy. This
view looked at the issues of health and disease much differently than
the medical establishment of that era. Cayce was decades ahead of his
time. We are only now beginning to realize the wisdom of his ways as
medical research verifies the success of the Cayce remedies in healing

migraines, Parkinson's disease, psoriasis, multiple sclerosis, and other chronic diseases for which modern medicine has not made the grade.

Another factor in Cayce's notoriety in the holistic health scene is that the source that spoke through Cayce often recommended natural remedies for the diseases being addressed. Significantly, this impetus came at a time in American history—the early twentieth century—that marked the rise in popularity of the allopathic, mechanistic, materialistic view of medicine. This modern medical model has led to our current health care crisis and to ads on TV and radio touting the value of the "new purple pill"—never mind the long list of possible side effects. There has to be a better way.

The Cayce Approach to Health

The majority of recorded readings were given specifically for the purpose of helping with personal health issues. The Cayce health readings addressed diseases not as distinct entities in and of themselves but rather by how they manifested in each individual. Yet, over the years certain general principles of health and healing became evident. Although the Cayce readings do not directly address animal health issues, the general health guidelines apply as much to the fitness of our four-legged friends as they do to our own well-being.

Let's look at how some of the fundamental concepts from the Cayce readings apply to our animal companions.

Holistic Medicine

Edgar Cayce's health philosophy is first and foremost a holistic view. The term "holistic" is used quite freely these days, and its meaning may have become somewhat unclear, especially as holistic medicine has hit the mainstream. To look at another being holistically is to affirm that there is more to the universe than meets the eye. As we covered in chapter 1, all sentient beings are made up of mental and spiritual aspects as well as the physical body. All three dimensions must be addressed for true healing.

Holistic therapies embrace the vitalist concept that has been abandoned by conventional medicine. The vitalists believe that there is a vital energy that animates the flesh. The Chinese call it Qi; the Japanese call it Ki; the doctors of India call it Prana; homeopaths call it the Vital Force; and chiropractors call it the Innate. It is this life force energy that is the difference between life and death, and it must be nourished for true health.

For the most part, it appears that the energy systems of animals mirror the human energy system. This comparison has most thoroughly been explored in the field of veterinary acupuncture. The ancient Chinese did use acupuncture on animals; however, they just used a handful of points and did not work out the meridian system as they did in people. The animal meridians have only recently been mapped out by Western veterinarians.

Individually Specific Care

In today's medical approach, individuals are grouped into disease categories and treated accordingly. The Cayce method, and that of holistic pet care in general, is much different. Cayce gave readings for individuals and treatment tailored to that particular person. Different individuals with the same disease may need different treatments.

The same disease acts upon each entity differently. Also, the same end product, or disease, may result from diverse causes. It is not sufficient to know the name of the disease; it is much more important to know the individual suffering from the particular affliction.

Since we do not have the psychic abilities of Edgar Cayce, holistic practitioners generally spend extra time with their patients. There are many methods for determining energetic disturbances, including Chinese pulse and tongue diagnoses, acupressure and muscle testing. We also generally get a detailed background of the patient from her caregiver. When we put all this information together, often a pattern emerges, allowing us to treat the root of the problem for that patient.

Let's look at arthritis. Different pets manifest arthritis differently. Some are worse in cold weather, some worse in damp weather; and for others, the weather has no effect. Some arthritic pets are in pain and others are simply stiff. Holistically speaking, each of these conditions requires a different approach. So from this perspective, I have never treated arthritis. I have treated many patients suffering from arthritis, but each is an individual, and the disease has no meaning unless discussed with respect to that particular patient.

The Body's Pharmacy

The Cayce philosophy honors the body's ability to heal itself. The body is viewed as containing its own pharmacy. Research bears this fact out. You may have heard of the placebo effect. This medical anomaly predicts that 30 percent of subjects treated with a sugar pill will improve—no matter what the disease is. High blood pressure, low blood pressure, allergies, etc., all can be alleviated by the patients' own bodies. It is considered a case of mind over matter, but it proves that our bodies can heal themselves if conditions are right. The goal of holistic therapies in pets is to produce the right conditions for an animal's body to heal itself. Obviously, the animal's belief system does not affect the results of therapy, so there must be other factors at work.

Dis-ease Prevention

According to the holistic concepts embraced by Cayce, health is considered to be more than simply the absence of disease. It is a state of well-being expressed as a vitality that resists disease. Health is a dynamic balance of internal and external forces. From this point of view, there is a broad spectrum of physical conditions ranging from perfect health to death. Dis-ease begins as an imbalance, which may go undetected by conventional means. If left untreated at this early stage, detectable disease will eventually result.

Have you ever had the experience of taking your pet to the veterinarian because he is not acting right only to be told after a battery of tests that there is nothing wrong. If your pet is having even mild symptoms, you know there is something wrong. The problem is that conventional testing and conventional wisdom do not recognize the disturbance until it becomes more serious. Most holistic approaches have ways of diagnosing and treating the imbalance before it develops into disease, not to mention advice on a healthy lifestyle to maintain health.

Personal Responsibility

Recipients of Cayce health readings were often directed to apply their own treatments and practices to help themselves regain or maintain health. This is an empowering idea, and one that flies in the face of current medical practice. In today's world, patients are often expected to shut up and do what the doctor says. Doctors, and unfortunately this includes many veterinarians, do not like to be bothered by patients/clients who ask a lot of questions. And yet, studies have shown that human patients who question their doctors and get involved in their health care decisions have far better outcomes than those who do not.

From my experience as a veterinarian, I feel strongly that the same is true of pets whose owners are active participants in the healing process of the animal. Holistic therapies in pets often require that owners roll up their sleeves and do their part. From making a special diet to physical therapy to acupressure, caretaker involvement is mandatory. When people come in expecting me to do all the work to "fix" their pet, they are often disappointed. The maintenance of health is a constant battle that cannot be won by periodic veterinary visits alone. At the very least, the caregiver must pay close attention to how the pet responds to treatments so the practitioner can modify his approach.

Disease Symptoms vs. Underlying Cause

Modern medicine is geared toward quick-fix symptom relief. "Eat whatever you like, just take this pill first." What a concept! For headaches you can take four pills per day or just one. And everybody knows that the minute you detect a fever, you should take something to suppress it. Why bother finding out what the problem is or maintaining a healthy lifestyle to avoid the problem in the first place?

The Cayce readings, like the holistic approach, target the underlying cause of the disease. Although it is sometimes necessary to relieve the suffering caused by symptoms, in general, symptoms are viewed as the body's response to the disease. Symptoms guide the holistic practitioner to the core issue causing the imbalance and sometimes symptoms are a legitimate response of the body.

For example, we often forget that no germ creates a fever. The body generates the increased temperature that occurs with infection. Why? Many germs can only survive at normal body temperature. The fever itself kills the invaders. A high body temperature also increases the efficacy of the immune system. Finally, a fever usually forces the individual to rest, which further helps the body regenerate. So what do we commonly do? At the first sign of fever, we take an aspirin to counteract our body's natural defenses so we can keep working. The end result is that the disease lingers.

The holistic Cayce approach not only works with the body's natural defenses to fight the disease, it addresses the issue of why the individual was susceptible to the sickness in the first place.

Natural Remedies

The holistic medical method honors the fact that Mother Nature has supplied us with much of what we need to get healthy and stay healthy. Given the side effects of conventional medicines, proper nutrition, herbs, and natural therapies are often the safest way to go.

Unfortunately, the term "natural" is quite a buzzword these days as more and more people are becoming interested in holistic treatments. When most of us think of natural remedies we think of herbs and vitamins. However, I have been seeing more and more synthetic compounds being labeled as "natural" to cash in on the holistic market. In fact, many "natural" vitamins are manufactured by pharmaceutical companies. Let's face it, ultimately everything comes from nature. The word "natural" has become almost meaningless.

Another matter to consider is the proper use of truly natural remedies. No remedy, whether natural or synthetic is without possible side effects. The right remedy must be applied to the right condition, and it takes some knowledge to do this properly. It is important to have any problem your pet may be facing properly diagnosed by a veterinarian. It is equally important to have any natural remedy administered by a practitioner who is trained in the use of such therapies in animals. Remember that anything that has the power to heal also has the power to harm, if misapplied. Death, too, is a "natural" process but this is obviously not the goal of holistic therapy.

An Integrative Approach

The Cayce readings acknowledge that there is validity to all therapeutic modalities. Cayce sometimes recommended strong medications or surgery as well as herbs and energy medicine. The proper therapy must be matched to the individual situation. This view is especially true in veterinary medicine where not only the condition and the animal must be assessed, but also the attitude and mindset of the caregiver.

Holistic therapies have much to offer and can treat many problems that modern medicine does not handle well. Chronic conditions such as arthritis are frequently treated successfully with acupuncture, herbs, and nutrition. Current treatments for such conditions are often accompanied by serious side effects.

At the same time modern diagnostics and treatments have their place. Diagnosing the disease is especially important in animals because they cannot tell us what is wrong and often instinctually hide their pain.

For example, a limping pet may have arthritis, a fracture, or a tumor. A simple X–ray can easily guide the practitioner to the proper therapy. There are natural therapies that address fractures, but most times surgery or casting makes more sense. God gave us the natural ability to come up with "unnatural" cures. I think of it as co–creating health.

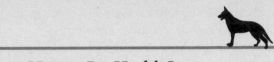

Unique Pet Health Issues

This chapter is not going to list suggestions for treatments or home remedies for specific problems. Since the same problem may have different causes in different individuals, it is best for each patient to be assessed and treated by a qualified animal practitioner. At the same time there are some general health guidelines that will benefit any pet.

Food for Thought

Let's begin by looking at our pets' diets. They say you are what you eat, and the same concept holds true for our pets. A healthy diet is the foundation for overall health. But what is a healthy diet for animals?

Commercial Diets

Take a critical look at your pet's food. Does it look appetizing to you? How did we ever get brainwashed into thinking that dry kibble or pre-digested canned foods are good for our pets. You might ask, "Well, what's the matter with it. It's pet food for goodness sake." There are a number of concerns I have about commercial pet foods.

First of all, what exactly are the ingredients? Look at the label. It says there is meat of some sort, usually beef, chicken, or lamb. But what is the quality of this meat? Did you know that there is no federal inspection of pet food processing? In many states it is considered OK to use meats that are unfit for human consumption. They call them the 4 Ds— Animals that arrive at the packing plant already dead, dying, diseased, or disabled. So, basically, they can cut diseased tissues and tumors off a carcass and throw it in the bin for pet foods. It's only pet food, right? I'm not saying that all pet foods contain these ingredients, but there is no way of knowing.

Another common ingredient in commercial diets is grain, such as corn, wheat, or rice. Many times this is the most abundant ingredient in the food. So, what's the matter with grain? It's good for you, right? Don't pets need carbohydrates? To answer these questions, look at the natural situation. What do our pet's counterparts in the wild eat? Wild members of the dog and cat families eat other animals. You don't see them grazing in the rice paddies for food. Now it is true that they eat some vegetation, but certainly carbohydrates are not the major part of their diets.

The fact is that carbohydrates are a cheap source of energy for foods. Unfortunately, I have seen evidence that the excessive amounts of carbohydrates in pet foods contribute to diabetes. I recently had a case where I could not regulate the glucose in a diabetic cat. We were giving large doses of insulin with no results. I had the owner switch the cat to a carbohydrate free natural diet, and within days we had the glucose under control. I also believe that the high level of carbohydrates in pet foods leads to obesity. It is the best explanation I can find for why a 100–pound Labrador Retriever gains weight on one cup of food per day.

I also have a problem with some of the additives they use in pet foods. Many foods contain artificial flavors and colors. These are unnatural chemicals that have no place in our pets' diets. How about preservatives? Did you know that the burger–type semi–moist foods are preserved with sugar? Imagine, there is so much sugar in them that bacteria can't survive. That doesn't sound very healthy.

One of the trickiest pet food ingredients to preserve is fat. Fat is an important nutrient for animals but it goes rancid quite easily when left out at room temperature. The most common fat preservative is ethoxyquin. Over the years, concerned pet owners have sought foods that are ethoxyquin free. This task is not as easy as it sounds. If a food company buys fat and adds ethoxyquin to preserve it, they must put ethoxyquin on the label. However, if the food company buys fat that already has ethoxyquin in it, they do not have to list the ingredient. So much for reading labels.

Of course, we do have some pet food companies that are adding healthy supplements to their foods. For example, there are ads for foods containing glucosamine for healthy joints. The problem is that there is great disparity in the quality of glucosamine supplements, and there is no way of assessing the quality from the label. Also, it is necessary to supply this supplement at an adequate dose to have the desired effect. I question whether pets really get enough from these foods.

There are also companies that tout that their pet foods contain essential fatty acids for a healthy coat. Unfortunately, essential fatty acids do not maintain their potency unless they are kept from exposure to open air and light. No dry pet food can keep this nutrient active. The food may have contained essential fatty acids when it left the factory but little if any of it makes it to your pet.

Both glucosamine and essential fatty acids are very important for proper nutrition, but they are best supplied to your pet in the form of a high quality supplement. Or better yet, feed your pet a natural diet, which automatically contains all the needed nutrients, even those we have yet to discover. We will look more closely at these topics shortly.

Commercial diets also fall short when it comes to the very form in which they are delivered to our pets. Cayce stressed the importance of eating slowly and chewing food thoroughly. Digestion begins in the mouth. Animals chew their food not just to break it into pieces that can be swallowed, but also to mix the food with saliva. Saliva contains enzymes that begin the digestive process before the food even reaches the stomach. Canned food is so mushy that pets don't have to chew it, and dry food comes in small kibble that many pets swallow whole. Wild dogs and cats eat raw food containing bones that have to be chewed. Thus, even the form of our pet foods bypasses the natural process of eating.

Finally with respect to commercial diets, look at the processing. Do wolves cook their food before eating? Have you ever seen a tiger light up a Bunsen burner? I don't think so. Wild animals eat their food raw, the way nature intended. Our pets, too, have evolved for millions of years on raw food. In fact, processed food is a recent development and has been fed to pets for only the past seventy years or so. So what's so bad about cooking the ingredients, it still contains all the same proteins, right? Well, not exactly. Heat denatures the proteins and destroys some other nutrients. One major ingredient that cooking destroys is the food's natural enzymes.

Every cell in the body contains enzymes. When an animal dies, the cellular enzymes release and dissolve the tissues. In medical terms this is called autolysis. When an animal eats raw foods it benefits from these naturally occurring enzymes because the normal diet helps digest itself. Cooked food contains no enzymes and is not digested and assimilated properly. This is why adding digestive enzymes to commercial pet foods can greatly benefit the health of our pets.

So, if we compare commercial diets to the natural diet that carnivores are meant to eat, we see that commercial diets do not measure up. Pet food companies start with questionable raw materials, add potential toxins, then process the nutrition out. Finally the food manufacturers try ineffectively to add back nutrients. Let's face it, pet foods are made more for our convenience than for pet nutrition. In fact, another reason many of our pets are overweight is that they are starved for nutrients, and we are feeding them empty calories. The alternative is to feed our pets the natural diet they were meant to eat.

Home Prepared Diets

So what is a natural diet for pets? How can an average pet owner make his pet's food? Surely only food companies know the secret to formulating a proper diet. Think about it, pets have been around for a long time before pet food manufacturers existed. Why do we not have the same concerns about feeding the human members of our families?

Before talking about what a natural diet is, let me explain what it is not. Feeding animals human food is not the same as feeding table scraps. The scraps from our tables usually include fat, cooked bones, and processed foods, all of which can cause serious health problems for our pets.

A natural diet for pets also does not mean feeding them only meat. Although dogs and cats are carnivores, their normal diet also includes raw bones, organ meat, such as liver, and shredded vegetables. The biggest problem with feeding only meat is that meat is high in phosphorus. It is extremely important to balance this phosphorus with the proper amount of calcium, which the animals normally get by eating raw bones.

There are two basic philosophies on making homemade pet diets. Dr.

Richard Pitcairn was a pioneer in holistic pet health and wrote one of the first books on the subject, *Natural Health for Dogs and Cats*. This book is a must for all pet owners. In it, Dr. Pitcairn gives information on pet diets and gives several recipes. Dr. Pitcairn meticulously researched these diets for proper balance. The problem is that he based his research on conventional concepts of pet nutrition. The biggest flaw is that these recipes are high in carbohydrates. The other drawback is the complexity of preparation with many supplements added. But, these diets can be cooked, so if you cannot bring yourself to feed raw meat, these recipes are for you.

Another approach to pet nutrition is to mimic nature and base the pet diet on what similar wild animals eat. This dietary philosophy is abbreviated BARF which stands for Bones And Raw Foods. A proponent of this diet is Dr. Ian Billinghurst from Australia. *Give Your Dog a Bone* is his book outlining the BARF diet. *Natural Nutrition for Dogs and Cats,* by Kymythy R. Schultze, is another good book on this subject.

The BARF diet is based on the concept that our pets are made to eat what their wild counterparts eat. Wild dogs, such as wolves, and wild cats, such as bobcats, eat raw meat and raw bones with some organ meat and shredded veggies that they get from the abdominal contents of their prey. As mentioned above, raw meat is much different than cooked meat. Raw is more nutritious than cooked for our pets.

Feeding raw meat always brings up the concern over bacteria and parasites. All I can say is that they do not seem to cause a problem for wild animals and they do not seem to bother pets either. Their digestive systems handle it just fine. For the past five years I have been feeding my own two dogs and four cats raw meat, mostly chicken and turkey, and have had no problems with bacterial infections. In fact, Louie, my Newfoundland mix, has been known to bury a chicken back, then dig it up the next day and eat it, with no deleterious effects.

Yes, I feed my dogs bones. It is true that cooked bones are very dangerous. They are brittle and break into sharp pieces, which can rip through a pet's intestines. The right raw bones, however, are a bird of a different feather. They can be easily digested by pets, and have been for millions of years.

When including vegetables in a pet's diet they need to be shredded, just like the kind found in the herbivore's stomach. The carnivore's digestive tract is shorter than that of an herbivore and therefore cannot handle whole vegetables. Shredded vegetables are very nutritious as part of a pet's diet.

Although vegetables are part of a pet's diet, it is not natural for dogs and cats to be vegetarians. Having said this, it is possible for dogs to thrive on a vegetarian diet if it is combined carefully. Cats on the other hand are obligate carnivores. There are certain nutrients found only in meat that cats must have to live.

The beauty of the BARF diet is that very few supplements are needed. That's the way it should be when you feed the pet what it is meant to eat. I recommend simply adding a natural multivitamin/mineral to the diet for good measure. Be sure to read a good book on the subject before starting your pet on the BARF diet.

Supplements

Closely related to the subject of a natural diet is the idea of using nutritional supplements. There are many different types of supplements. Some are meant as an additive to help balance the diet and others are aimed at specific pet problems. Let's look at some useful dietary supplements.

Vitamins—I think that the use of vitamin supplements in general is a good idea, especially for those who feed their animal companions commercial foods.

For one thing, the government determines the proper level of vitamins in food to be the amount necessary to prevent deficiency disease. In most cases, this is less than the amount needed for optimal health under normal conditions and much less than what is required during times of stress.

This minimal amount of vitamins is added to the food before processing. The heat of processing destroys many vitamins. In the case of dry foods, much of the vitamin content that remains is quickly lost if the product is not consumed soon after manufacture. Finally, minerals are often added in forms that are not absorbed by the body.

But if pet foods contain such poor nourishment, why is it that all our pets are not dropping over dead from malnutrition? The reason is that vitamin deficiencies more commonly cause a state of chronic, poor health. Poorly fed animals are more prone to infectious disease and parasites. This condition eventually progresses to more serious problems such as skin disease, arthritis, kidney disease, and cancer.

All pets can benefit from vitamin supplements; however, the form the supplements take is important. Most vitamin supplements are manufactured synthetically by pharmaceutical companies. Synthetic vitamins are slightly different chemically than are natural vitamins and are not utilized by the body as effectively.

Also, most common vitamin supplements are formulated under the presumption that we know everything there is to know about nutrition. This is not a safe assumption. Scientists are discovering "new" phytochemical nutrients every day. Researchers are also just starting to realize the importance of these nutrients to good health.

The best way for animals to get the nutrients they need is from whole foods. This is because vitamins need the phytochemicals found in whole foods to be fully active. These vitamin cofactors greatly enhance the usefulness of the vitamins to the body.

For general dietary support, I recommend "Standard Process" brand nutritional supplements. These supplements are made by removing the fiber and water from organically grown foods. The nutritional components from various foods are then combined to provide a balance of natural nutrients.

Glucosamine—One important nutrient that we touched on earlier is glucosamine. Glucosamines are natural compounds that are a combination of glucose and the amino acid, glutamine. Glucosamines, in turn, are the building blocks for connective tissues, joint tissues, and intestinal lining tissue.

Combinations of glucosamine molecules with various proteins form the matrix between the cells of the body, holding them together. These compounds are also responsible for the gelatinous nature of cartilage. They allow cartilage to hold water, which gives this tissue its slippery shock–absorbing quality.

Research has shown that taking glucosamine supplements can help protect weakened joints. In fact, they can actually help deformed, arthritic joints rebuild healthy tissue.

One human study compared the use of ibuprofen with glucosamine in arthritic patients. At first, ibuprofen was more effective at reducing joint inflammation and pain. After a longer period, though, the glucosamine outperformed the ibuprofen by repairing the joint cartilage and decreasing inflammation.

Glucosamine supplements can be used to benefit many degenerative conditions such as osteoarthritis, hip dysplasia, spinal arthritis, and other joint problems.

Because of glucosamine's importance as a building block for the intestinal lining, it has also been proven to help with cases of inflammatory bowel disease, an intestinal disorder of animals similar to Crohn's disease in people.

Glucosamines are very valuable to the health of our pets. However, not all glucosamine supplements are equal. The quality of this nutrient depends on how it is processed. Also, its beneficial effects are dose dependent.

I am familiar with Glyco–Flex and have found it very helpful in aiding arthritic joints. This product is made from Green–Lipped Mussel, an edible shellfish, which is a rich source of amino acids, vitamins, naturally chelated minerals, fatty acids, and nucleic acids, as well as glucosamine compounds.

Essential Fatty Acids—Many skin disorders and other health problems of pets are caused by a lack of proper fats in the diet. In order to supplement these nutrients correctly, we need a little background in this oily area of nutrition.

Fats and oils are composed of fatty acids. There are many types of fatty acids, but the important types are the Omega 3s and Omega 6s. These are considered the essential fatty acids (EFAs) because the body cannot produce them and must get them from food.

EFAs play a part in almost every function in the body. They govern growth, mental states, and are even a key factor in the burning of food to produce energy.

EFA molecules are very fragile. That is why Mother Nature packages them in hard seeds such as flax, sesame, and sunflower. The seed shells protect the EFAs from heat, light and oxygen, which destroy the nutrients.

Commercial oils from the grocery store are highly processed. This processing involves adding chemicals and bleaching the oils to improve the shelf life. The oils are then heated to frying temperature, all of which destroys the natural EFAs.

These are not only the oils we consume but are also the "nutrients" added to pet foods. Any EFAs that may be left in the pet foods are often rancid by the time the pet consumes them because they are not protected from the air. This is why most pets (and people) can benefit from EFA supplementation.

Another cause of EFA deficiency is the consumption of harmful fats. These are the hydrogenated and saturated fats found in margarine and processed foods. EFAs compete with these useless fats in the body, and if the EFAs do not win, the body loses.

Now that we have established the need for adding EFAs to the diet, we can open the debate over the proper ratio of Omega 3s and Omega 6s to be supplemented. Too much of one can lead to a deficiency of the other. Animals tend to be more deficient in Omega 3s because they are more easily destroyed. Supplementing Omega 3s and 6s at a 2:1 ratio seems to be widely accepted.

Sources high in Omega 3s include flax seed oil and fish oils. However, feeding theses oils exclusively can lead to a deficiency in Omega 6s. The use of sunflower oil can help maintain the balance.

Again, it is important that these oils be cold processed and stored in light-resistant bottles to keep their nutritional value. Your local health food store or veterinarian is likely to have what your pet needs.

Lack of sufficient EFAs tend to manifest in the skin first because the vital internal organs take what they need first. The skin is the first to lose the oils and the last to get them. The deficiency can lead to dry, flaky, itchy skin.

Supplementing EFAs may also improve arthritis, obesity, immune function, gastrointestinal disorders, kidney disease, and cardiovascular dysfunction. Older animals commonly show an increase in energy while young animals recover more quickly from fatigue and heal faster. I have had much success with a product called "Dream Coat."

Research has shown that animals often have trouble absorbing the oils in their diet. Adding digestive enzymes to the diet can increase the absorption of EFAs by 200 percent. I recommend "Prozyme" as a digestive enzyme supplement.

Vaccinations

Vaccinations are the conventional veterinarian's weapon for preventive medical care. In fact, vaccinations are often the only tool for disease prevention. The struggle to maintain health becomes a battle against disease instead of a process of aiding the body to function at its highest level.

The idea behind vaccines is to give the immune system a taste of a germ so the disease fighting mechanism will react to the unwanted invader when needed. This concept actually originated in ancient China as inoculations. The Chinese took the discharge from a sick individual and introduced it onto the mucous membranes of a healthy person in order to instill immunity. It is important to note that only one disease was inoculated and that it was introduced into the body in the same way that the natural infection would invade.

The current practice of vaccinating animals is significantly different in many ways. Vaccines are administered by injection, while the diseases they are meant to prevent are naturally spread through contact with the mucous membranes. A natural infection first encounters the immune system through the lymphoid tissue in the mouth, nose, and throat, such as the tonsils. This triggers the immune system the way nature intended. When the vaccine is injected, the stimulus bypasses this important step, and the immune system is ambushed.

Current dog and cat vaccines also contain as many as seven different diseases. Let's face it, it's the American way. "The more the merrier. Let's supersize that vaccine." Well, this is a very abnormal situation. How often does an animal catch six different viruses at the same time? Add to this, the fact that some veterinarians vaccinate pets that are not in a completely healthy state. It's just more convenient to go ahead and give the shot while the pet is at the office being treated for an ear infection or allergy or whatever. Even the vaccine label says to vaccinate only healthy pets.

To add insult to injury, we veterinarians, in our quest to prevent diseases in pets, have for decades been following the vaccine manufacturers' recommendations for administering vaccinations on a yearly basis for the life of the animal. The practice of annual vaccination is based on research done in 1962. Needless to say, vaccine technology has come a long way in the past few decades.

Recent studies show that the antibodies produced by administering most of the current dog and cat distemper vaccines remain at protective levels for at least three years, in adult animals. This fact has been in the veterinary literature for years now. Still the vaccine producers have the label recommendation of yearly boosters. This puts the veterinarian in a tough position.

The reason the recommendation remains, and the biggest argument against the use of antibody titers, is that high antibody levels do not guarantee immunity. There is more to the immune system than antibodies. Yet, the antibody level is the test used as the criterion for revaccinating veterinarians themselves for rabies. If this test is good enough to guide the protection of people who are at risk, from rabies, then it ought to be the standard for guiding the use of vaccines in animals. It is true that a high antibody titer does not guarantee immunity. Of course, vaccinating yearly does not guarantee immunity either.

The test that the vaccine companies rely on to establish the efficacy of their vaccines is called a challenge study. They vaccinate a group of animals, then challenge the animals by exposing them to the disease one year later. This proves that the vaccine is good for at least one year. But that's as far as the pharmaceutical companies go. They do not challenge the subjects again two or three or four years later. Since they are only sure the vaccines are good for one year, they recommend yearly boosters.

So, our current veterinary preventive medical program involves si-multaneously introducing multiple disease elements into the body in an abnormal way, assaulting the pet's immune system, and repeating that process more frequently than needed. My question is, "What is the overall effect of this on the animal's immune system?"

The immune system performs the very important function of pro-tecting the body from abnormal conditions. It recognizes, seeks out, and destroys germs that invade the body. The immune system also pro-tects the body against cancer cells. A properly functioning immune sys-tem is imperative for life.

There are two basic ways that the immune system can malfunction. With the first type of failure, the immune system becomes underactive, which allows infections to take hold and make our pets ill. Also, an underactive immune system cannot filter out abnormal cells. This is an important point.

The body is made up of trillions of cells. As these cells reproduce, mutations occur. It is by this mechanism that every day, a normal body produces at least one cancer cell. Why aren't all our pets dying from cancer? Because the immune system swoops in and destroys these ab-normal cells before the cancer can take hold. However, an unhealthy immune system can't do its job properly, and cancer can be the result. Of course, there are many factors that go into the formation of cancer, including a possible genetic predisposition and toxins in the food, wa-ter, and environment. The body's immune system does play a key role in the prevention of cancer.

So, a weak immune system is hazardous to health. At the same time, the second type of immune system malfunction, where it becomes over-active, can be just as dangerous. If the immune system becomes over-sensitive, it will overreact to normal stimuli or even seek and destroy normal tissue.

When the immune system overreacts to normal stimuli, we call the result an allergy. Think about it, if your pet is allergic to wheat, the problem is not the wheat, but the animal's immune system, which is reacting to something that it should ignore. Yet, what is the conven-tional approach to allergies? Well, we test to see what the pet is allergic to and then we try to either eliminate the allergen from the animal's environment, or we try to desensitize the immune system with allergy shots. Even if either of these approaches is successful, it is usually not long before the animal begins to react to something new because the pet still has a sick immune system.

An even more dangerous conventional treatment for allergies is to pump the pet full of steroids in an attempt to partially shut down the immune system. This quick fix weakens the entire immune system, and I already mentioned what can happen when the immune system is weakened. Remember, inflammatory bowel disease and recurrent ear infections can also be related to allergies.

As I mentioned, an overactive immune system will sometimes destroy normal tissue. For some reason the immune system occasionally becomes sensitized to certain cells of the body and sees them as foreign invaders. The immune system then does what any good immune system would do, it destroys the supposed intruder. This condition is referred to as an autoimmune disease.

The immune system may attack red blood cells, causing anemia as with immune mediated hemolytic anemia; it can attack platelets, causing bleeding as in immune mediated thrombocytopenia; it can even attack the skin, causing blisters as in pemphigus. You may not have heard of these diseases, but did you know that hypothyroidism, diabetes, certain forms of arthritis, and even cruciate ligament ruptures have been linked to autoimmune disease. The origin of most of these immune system troubles is rarely discovered.

Coincidentally, recent studies have linked potentially fatal diseases to vaccines. These afflictions include a specific kind of cancer in cats and certain autoimmune diseases in dogs. Plus, we are all aware of the occasional allergic reaction to vaccines.

I will grant that these diseases that have been directly linked to vaccines are somewhat uncommon. However, there may be many more diseases brought on by vaccines that have yet to be associated due to their insidious nature. Many veterinarians agree that cancer, allergies, and autoimmune diseases are more common these days than ever before. This increase in immune system–related problems corresponds

with the increase in popularity of current, excessive vaccination proto-
cols. Could it be that our own preventive medical programs are actually
preventing health?

I think it is time to treat vaccinating as the medical procedure it is.
The decision on how frequently to vaccinate an animal should be made
on an individual basis. It should be based on a risk benefit ratio. Also,
the decision should be based on blood titers.

I am not against vaccines. On the contrary, having worked at a humane society for five years, I have seen firsthand just how important
vaccines are in the reduction of such deadly pet diseases as rabies, distemper, and parvo. I am, however, against the current overuse of vaccines in our pets. Although puppies and kittens do need regular vaccine
boosters to insure immunity, I currently vaccinate most adult animals
every three years for distemper and parvo. This general recommendation is adjusted on an individual basis, depending on risk factors.

I also recommend that you do not vaccinate your pet for irrelevant
diseases. For example, many canine distemper combination vaccines
contain a Leptospirosis strain that is no longer being spread in the wild.
It doesn't make sense to include a useless component in the vaccine.
Recently, an updated version of the Leptospirosis component has been
developed. If you live in an area where Leptospirosis is found, be sure
to have your pet vaccinated with the proper strain. If this infection is
not important in your region, do not vaccinate your pet for this disease.

Canine Coronavirus is another vaccine of dubious usefulness. I have
heard Coronavirus described as a vaccine waiting for a disease. The
virus is said to cause diarrhea although it has been found in the stool of
healthy pets. If Coronavirus does cause diarrhea, the pet almost always
gets over the disease in a few days with no treatment. Is it worthwhile
to vaccinate for such a disease just because we can? My answer is "No."

Lyme disease is a debilitating disease spread by ticks. The Lyme disease vaccine can be equally dangerous. Some dogs actually develop
symptoms of the disease after being vaccinated. If you live in an area
where Lyme disease is common, then consider the vaccine. If this disease is not common in your region, do not vaccinate your dog. No
matter which situation applies to you, if your dog is exposed to a tick

infested area, then use a product to repel or kill ticks. This strategy will help protect your pet from Lyme disease as well as the many other diseases that are spread by ticks.

For cats, remember that the Feline Leukemia Virus is spread from cat to cat by direct contact. If you have a strictly indoor cat that is never exposed to other cats, it does not need the Leukemia vaccine. All cats should be tested for this disease to be sure of their status, but the vaccine is for cats at risk of exposure to other cats of unknown disease condition.

Rabies, on the other hand is a serious disease with human health implications. Our pets are often an interface between wild animals that carry the life-threatening disease and us. Both dogs and cats should receive this vaccine as required by law. I recommend that the rabies and distemper vaccines not be given at the same time. Wait at least two weeks between vaccines to allow each to do its job.

It is important to realize that reducing the frequency of vaccination does not negate the need for yearly examinations of your pet. Especially in this day and age, pets need annual wellness exams. Remember that our pets age about seven times faster than we do. A yearly examination for them is equivalent to us being examined every seven years.

There are likely to be many new vaccines developed for dogs and cats in the near future. Now more than ever it is important to consider each vaccine carefully. It simply does not make sense to vaccinate every animal for every disease every year.

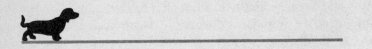

Specific Holistic Pet Therapies

Holistic therapies for pets have become more and more popular in recent years. The same techniques used on people can be applied to our pets; however, some are more readily adapted than others. From energy therapies such as Homeopathy, Reiki and Qi Gong to physical manipulations such as chiropractic and acupuncture to Eastern and Western herbal therapies, pets are benefiting from many alternative medical modalities. Let's take a look at some commonly available holistic pet therapies.

Traditional Chinese Medicine

The term Eastern medicine is used to denote the concepts of traditional Chinese medicine or TCM. TCM is a combination of practices and theories formalized into a system of medicine by the Chinese Taoists thousands of years ago. (Incidentally, the word "Tao" can be translated as "The Way" just as early Christians considered themselves to be followers of "The Way.") For the ancient Chinese, health care was a way of life. Diet, exercise, massage, meditation, sleep patterns, work patterns, herbs, and acupuncture were all integrated to balance the body through the external and internal cycles of life.

Just like Edgar Cayce, the ancient Chinese had a much different way of looking at the body than we currently do in the West. Chinese doctors did not have blood work, X-rays or other sophisticated diagnostic tests. These ancient physicians were armed with their five senses, astounding reasoning powers, experience and intuition. They were so in touch with their bodies and with nature that they were able to develop an intricate medical model that has stood the test of time. To understand their way of thinking we must let go of what we "know" about the workings of our bodies.

Watch the news. What experts "know" about health and medicine changes almost on a daily basis. Margarine is healthier than butter, then it isn't. Exposure to the sun causes skin cancer, then it stops it. What about the hormone replacement therapy farce? Each new study contradicts the last. In light of the state of modern medicine, the simple approach to health encompassed by TCM makes more and more sense.

Today, TCM is one of the most commonly employed holistic philosophies in veterinary medicine. Acupuncture is by far the most familiar holistic therapy used by veterinarians. There are currently four different institutions offering certification courses for veterinarians in the United

States, including two at universities. There are also several training courses for the use of Chinese herbs in pets. Given the popularity of TCM, it will be helpful to explore some of the basic concepts of this healing art.

Qi—Qi (pronounced "chee") is considered to be the life force energy. It is the force that keeps the body going. Qi is what separates the living from the dead. It has both structural and functional qualities. It is matter on the verge of becoming energy, and energy on the verge of materializing. Thousands of years after the Chinese understood this relationship, Einstein made us aware of it in the West with the formula "$E=mc^2$." This mathematical equation proves that energy (E) and matter, or mass (m), are fundamentally made up of the same material.

Qi is that substance from which all physical form is composed. Qi is also the energy that flows in a cyclic, orderly, predetermined course throughout the channels of the body, allowing for normal functioning of organs and tissues.

In TCM, health is the state of harmonious flow of Qi in the channels, organs, and tissues of the body. Disease is caused by the interruption in the flow of Qi. Any time an organ is not functioning properly, as in kidney failure, or a limb is not moving freely, as in arthritis, we can say there is a disturbance of Qi.

Yin and Yang—Another important TCM medical concept is the idea of yin and yang. The thought is that Qi (matter and energy) is expressed in the physical world as the interplay between relative opposites: darkness vs. light, feminine vs. masculine, rest vs. activity. All of creation is a result of the sacred dance of yin and yang.

The Chinese consider that all things have two aspects, a yin aspect and a yang aspect. There is no absolute yin or yang. We all know that even a real he-man has a feminine side. Any yin or yang aspect can be further divided into yin and yang, just as when a magnet is cut in half, two new magnets are created, each with a north and a south pole. Yin and yang are mutually dependent upon each other. The term "high" has no meaning without the concept of "low." Yin and yang control each other like a healthy marriage where the husband and wife balance each other. Yin and yang transform into each other as day turns to night and night turns back to day again.

All diagnosis and treatment in TCM may be reduced to the concept of yin and yang. Health is simply a state of harmonious balance between yin and yang. Disease is a condition of imbalance between yin and yang. The elderly cat that craves heat is probably lacking yang whereas the hyperactive dog may have too much yang.

Chinese Organs—As you might imagine, the Chinese had a different way of looking at the organs of the body than modern medicine does. Like the Cayce concept that every cell has consciousness, the Chinese consider that each organ has consciousness. The Chinese assigned different functions to the organs than are thought of in the West. In fact, in TCM the organs are not seen so much as physical structures as they are collections of functions.

Channels (Meridians)—There are fourteen main acupuncture channels which act as pathways for the flow of Qi along which lie the acupuncture points. The term *channel* is preferred because a meridian is an imaginary line, and the Chinese in no way considered the channels of energy to be imaginary.

These channels link the exterior of the body to the internal organs. There exists a complex cross-linking of channels. Each channel is named for the TCM organ to which it is most strongly associated. Qi flows through the channels in a particular direction, and flows from one channel to another via connecting pathways.

Acupuncture Points—Acupuncture points are discrete areas on the surface of the body that have unique features. These points have higher than normal numbers of nerve endings, blood vessels, and inflammatory cells. They are also areas of lower electrical resistance, meaning that electricity flows more readily at these areas. All of these features combine to amplify any stimulation of these points. The Chinese considered the acupuncture points as inlets to the channels. Through these inlets, the Qi of the body can be manipulated

Acupuncture—Acupuncture is one part of the TCM system. Acupuncture therapy involves the use of very fine needles to stimulate acupuncture points and induce a healing response. It has been used as a medical system in China for five thousand years.

Acupuncture has been used on animals for twenty–five hundred years. In fact the Chinese had the first medical practitioners that specialized on animals complete with their medical tests. So the world's first veterinarians were Chinese acupuncturists. Acupuncture is the most clinically tested form of medical treatment on earth. Even modern studies have shown that it works for many conditions.

According to TCM theory acupuncture manipulates the Qi of the body and rebalances the energy system to aid the body in healing itself. From the Western standpoint, acupuncture stimulates nerves that can block pain perception. Studies have also shown that acupuncture can be used to cause the release of hormones, including cortisone, as well as endorphins, which are the body's own morphine compounds. Acupuncture can reduce muscle spasms, increase circulation, and strengthen the immune system.

Acupuncture can help in the treatment of arthritis, kidney failure, liver failure, hyperthyroidism, asthma, back and joint injuries, vomiting, diarrhea, and reproductive problems. It can be used to help the treatment of seizures and even improve the quality of life for cancer patients. When used properly, this holistic approach does not cause serious side effects as drugs often do, although if desired, acupuncture can be used in conjunction with conventional therapies.

The biggest concern that most people have about veterinary acupuncture is that the needles will cause pain. In my experience, the patient rarely feels the needle. During a treatment I'm more concerned about the possibility that the patient may decide to remove a needle with his mouth and then swallow it. In reality, the biggest obstacle to this treatment is calming the pet enough to lie still while the needles work their magic. If the animal fidgets, often the needles fall out, which is not harmful but just not very helpful.

One of the most remarkable acupuncture cases I've seen is a little guinea pig named Betty. Betty had been dropped by the kids. Her spine was not broken but was injured to the point that she could not use her rear legs. She was treated conventionally with large doses of cortisone by her vet. I saw her one week after the injury. There was very little improvement in her condition. Her back legs were almost completely paralyzed.

I had never done acupuncture on a guinea pig before but the owner and I figured we had nothing to lose. I treated her at about 8:30 p.m. The owner called at 9:00 a.m. the next day. She told us that she reached into the cage to give Betty her medicine and the little rascal ran away from her. And Betty never looked back. Just one acupuncture treatment cured her condition.

I have to admit that this was an exceptional case. The two keys to the great outcome are that first of all it was an acute injury and secondly we treated it early.

A more common case is that of Grettle, a Doberman, who first came to me when she was nine years old. She was crippled in the rear legs due to severe arthritis of the hips. This condition had been going on for years. Grettle had been treated conventionally with the usual anti-inflammatory medications. Finally even cortisone was no longer helping her and her owners decided to try acupuncture as a last resort before putting her to sleep.

By the fourth weekly treatment Grettle's owner noticed that she was getting around better, and by the eighth treatment, she was keeping up with her younger sister. Grettle received acupuncture treatments every four to six weeks for two years before her body finally gave out. Those were two years of high quality life that Grettle's owner greatly appreciated.

Chinese Herbology—Another facet of TCM is Chinese Herbology. The development of this medical art has paralleled the progress of acupuncture. For millennia Chinese doctors have accumulated knowledge about the effects of the plants around them on the body.

The Chinese used many of the same herbs for healing as we do in the West. Ginger, licorice, and ginseng are shared as herbal remedies East and West. The difference between Chinese herbs and Western herbs is not so much the plants used as it is how those plants are used. First of all, Chinese herbs are utilized within the traditional Chinese medical model of organ function and energy balance.

Each herb used by the Chinese is characterized by the direction it tends to move energy, by how it affects the temperature of the body, what organ function it influences and what channels it enters. With this system the Chinese can pinpoint the effects that their remedies will have on the patient.

The Chinese also often use combinations of herbs for their synergistic effects. It is not uncommon to have ten or more herbs in a particular herbal formula. The use of herbal blends minimizes the possible side effects of individual substances.

A final difference between Western and Eastern herbs is that Chinese herbal medicine utilizes animal products such as turtle shell and deer antler as well as plants. So in the strictest sense, not all Chinese herbs are actually herbs.

Even today, the Chinese feel that this gentle, natural approach to healing is much safer than conventional medications for many ailments including cancer, skin conditions, internal organ problems, arthritis, and other chronic degenerative diseases. Many Chinese herbs can be used safely on our pets as well. But, be sure to consult a practitioner familiar with the use of herbs in animals.

Kerry is a five-year-old greyhound. He was a real mess when I first met him two months ago. He had large areas of hair loss all over his body and his skin was red and hot to the touch. All four of his paws were swollen with draining sores. His skin condition began after he was put on prednisone for his inflammatory bowel disease. He would not eat unless he got the medicine. Just before his digestive problems, he had an inflammation of both of his eyes. The interesting thing about this case is that all of Kerry's problems began right after he received his annual vaccines.

From a TCM standpoint, Kerry was diagnosed with liver fire invading the stomach. He was put on a mixture of Chinese herbs to cool the fire and support the liver. By the four-week progress exam, Kerry's skin was a normal pink color and back to a normal temperature. His feet were still very sore, but his attitude was much brighter. I changed his herbs to support his digestion and we began to taper down his prednisone dose.

Now, four weeks later his prednisone dose is cut to one quarter the amount and his appetite is still great. His feet are still sore though and we may have to resort to antibiotics to help his body clear the infection.

Chiropractic

The science of chiropractic manipulations was developed in the late 1800s. This healing modality is based on maintaining proper spinal alignment. Many of us are familiar with the use of chiropractic adjustments to treat back pain. The fact is that chiropractic was originally meant as a modality that addressed overall health.

The basic principle of chiropractic is that proper nerve flow to and from the body's organs and muscles is essential for their proper functioning. All of the nerves to the trunk and limbs of the body branch from the spinal cord, which is encased in the bony spine. In the course of normal activity the vertebrae of the spine can be jostled out of their proper positions. Add to this the rigors of athletic performance or the trauma of injuries and you can see how a pet's spine can become bent out of shape. Even minute misalignments in the spinal vertebrae can cause swelling that impinges on the nerves to the body. Spinal adjustments realign the spinal column, which allows for proper nerve flow to and from the organs and tissues of the body. This process underscores the importance of chiropractic to good overall health.

The Cayce readings stress the importance of maintaining proper spinal alignment. Although he often recommended osteopathic manipulations, Cayce did at times suggest chiropractic adjustments. There are no readily available courses for veterinarians to learn osteopathy but there is a comprehensive course in veterinary chiropractic. This 160 hour course is open to both veterinarians and chiropractors. Much is gained by both professions by the exchange of ideas. Veterinary chiropractic is becoming more popular and widely accepted as pet guardians and veterinarians witness the benefits of this therapy.

Allison is a four-year-old Irish Setter. Her life as a show dog requires her to walk around the ring with her head up, looking at her handler. This abnormal posture had led to her developing a slight hitch in her gait, which is unacceptable for a show dog. Regular spinal adjustments cleared up her lameness and she soon returned to the ring, winning ribbons.

Homeopathy

Homeopathy is a specific form of holistic medicine and the two terms are not synonymous. Homeopathy is a system of medicine that was developed about two hundred years ago by a German physician named Samuel Hahnemann. It is a system of treatment based on the use of natural remedies that in minute doses produce symptoms similar to those of the disease being treated, thus triggering the body's own immune response.

The basic premise of homeopathy is that all disease originates on the energetic level. So first there is a disturbance of the Vital Force. This imbalance then manifests physically as symptoms. Because the cause of disease is energetic, in order to eradicate disease it must be treated on the energetic level. Treating disease on the physical level with drugs or surgery only suppresses the disturbance, which will continue to develop and eventually erupt as a new set of symptoms.

Homeopathic care means treating a disease based on the symptoms it causes in the particular individual. The first homeopaths did thousands of experiments on human volunteers. A subject was given a natural compound until he developed symptoms. This process, called a proving, provided lists of symptoms caused by hundreds of compounds. Homeopathy literally means like cures like. Thus if a patient develops certain symptoms, the disease can be cured by treating him with a remedy which in a healthy individual causes similar symptoms.

This concept is in contrast to allopathy, which is a term for treating disease with a medical system using any principle other than like cures like. So, if a pet has a fever and it is treated with an anti-inflammatory such as aspirin or even a cooling herb, this is allopathy. For example, an allopathic treatment for a burn of the hand is to run cold water over it. The homeopathic cure for that same condition is to run very warm water over your hand—like cures like. Try it the next time you get a burn. You'll find the wound will blister less and heal faster.

Homeopathic remedies are produced by diluting and re-diluting a natural substance over and over. With each dilution the solution is shaken vigorously. Many homeopathic remedies are diluted to the point that not one molecule of the original remedy remains. This is why conventional medicine cannot accept that homeopathy has any physical effect on the body. Only the energy of the substance, which is transmitted in the fluid, is administered to the patient.

Of course, it is not the dilution that makes a remedy homeopathic but rather the way the remedy is used. To be homeopathic, the symptoms of the remedy must be matched to the symptoms of the individual patient. By definition, the use of multiple remedies at the same time for a condition such as arthritis is not homeopathy. Different pets manifest arthritis differently. Using combination remedies to try to cover all the various expressions of arthritis is not homeopathy and will likely suppress the disease, causing it to manifest in some other way.

Homeopathy is quite effective at treating many physical and mental disturbances, even conditions that cannot be adequately diagnosed conventionally. There is a formal course available for veterinarians to learn how to apply the principles of homeopathy to pets. This therapy is very difficult to apply to pets because they cannot directly relay their symptoms to the doctor. It takes a seasoned veterinary homeopath to use this method successfully on animal patients.

Butch was four months old when he contracted parvo. This is a very deadly virus of dogs, which causes vomiting and bloody diarrhea. The typical parvo case requires seven to ten days in the hospital on IV fluids and antibiotics. Even with aggressive treatment, some of these dogs die.

Butch was evaluated homeopathically. The same remedy would not be appropriate for every case of parvo. I took into consideration such factors as the color and smell of the stool, the degree of thirst, the mental attitude, and the frequency and color of the vomit. After just three doses of the right remedy and no fluids or antibiotics, Butch was released from the hospital with no symptoms.

There are many holistic therapies available for pets these days. I have described the most popular techniques that are becoming more accepted in the veterinary community. These modalities have formal training programs for veterinarians, as well as certification processes and organizations to oversee the practice of the various healing arts. Be sure to check the credentials of the practitioner you choose for your pet. Further information about holistic veterinary care organizations can be found on the Web site of Complementary and Alternative Veterinary Medicine at www.altvetmed.com.

Edgar Cayce advocated the use of natural physical, herbal, and energy healing methods, such as the ones mentioned above. Our animal companions are such an important part of our lives, and we want to keep them healthy and happy for their natural lifespan. The holistic approach can assure this goal. In the words of an ancient Chinese medical book, the *Nei Jing*, "Maintaining order rather than correcting disorder is the ultimate principle of wisdom. To cure disease after it has happened is like digging a well when one already feels thirsty or forging weapons after the war has already begun."

Your pet's well-being is in your hands. Pay attention to subtle changes and get involved in your pet's health care. As your animal friends reach their golden years prepare yourself for the weakening of the body associated with aging as well as the impending transition.

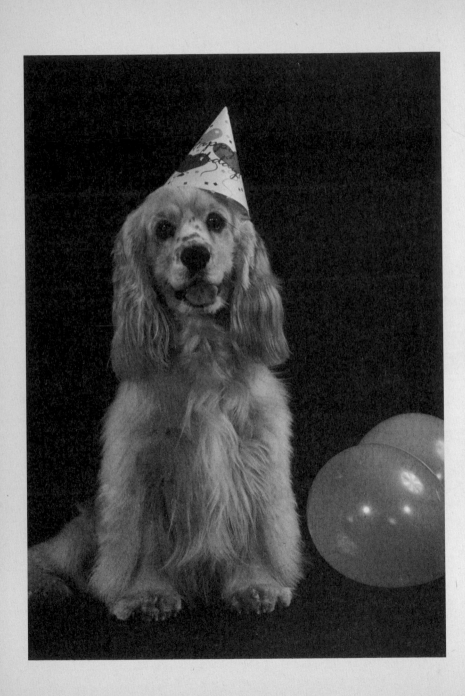

CHAPTER

6

THE END

... there is no death, only the transition from the physical to the spiritual plane.
                                                        136-36

It is a cold, hard reality that death is a part of life. No *body* is getting out of this thing alive. Because our pets have a much shorter lifespan than we do, our animal friends have a lot to teach us about the dying process, the mystery of crossing over, and the emotional state associated with those loved ones who are left behind.

Senior Pets

It is sometimes difficult for us to watch a beloved pet grow beyond the prime of her life. She may begin to develop chronic health problems. Crippling arthritis, debilitating kidney failure, and insidious cancer are all too common plights for today's companion animals. It is a lesson to us all that our animal friends face these afflictions with dignity and courage.

As our veterinary medical technology advances, we veterinarians find we are faced with more and more patients of advanced years. In fact the term "senior" has been designated to refer to that age at which there is a progressive decline in physical condition, organ function, mental function, and immunity—a state of affairs that many of us can relate to.

The concept of senior pet care involves providing for the specialized needs of aging pets. This effort is based on two ideas: first, that there are basic differences in the specific diseases, behavior problems, and nutritional needs of older animals; second, that prevention and early treatment of medical problems can greatly increase the longevity and quality of life of a senior pet.

Your pet does not have to be old and creaky to be considered a senior. In general, any pet over seven years old is a senior. Of course, some large breeds of dogs, such as Great Danes and Mastiffs, have shorter life spans and are considered senior at about five years. Other genetic factors can also cause a pet to age prematurely and need special care at an early age.

Treating your pet holistically can keep him healthier longer. We have explored the importance of a holistic lifestyle for your pet, and of course, maintenance of this way of life during the senior years goes without saying. At the same time, there are conventional means of assuring your companion's health. A truly holistic approach to aging honors the importance of diagnostic tests to keep abreast of your pet's health condition.

Many veterinarians have adopted senior pet programs that focus on pet owner education, disease prevention, and the early detection of medical conditions. In this way, the prognosis is better, and numerous treatment options still exist.

Studies have shown that many older pets may be suffering from conditions that are not readily apparent. Animals frequently hide their pain, and symptoms of many diseases are difficult to detect in the early stages. Often, people notice changes in their pets and chalk it up to old age, not realizing that treatment is available. Yet, if caught in the early stages, these conditions can be treated much more effectively, whether using conventional or alternative means.

For these reasons, it is best that pet owners become proactive in the care of their senior pets. I recommend that all senior pets have a complete physical exam every six months. I also advocate that once per year these older animals receive special tests. This yearly senior exam should include such tests as chest X-rays, blood chemistry profile, complete blood count (CBC), T-4 (thyroid hormone level), urinalysis, and tonometry (glaucoma test).

All of this testing may seem extreme. How many of us would subject ourselves to such diagnostics on a yearly basis. The point is that unlike us, our pets cannot let us know when they are having a problem. We usually must rely on tests for answers. Also, because they age about seven times faster than we do, yearly testing for them is like us being tested every seven years. Taking action before problems become obvious is the best way to keep your senior pet healthy and happy.

It is important to realize that aging alone does not cause symptoms. There are, however, age-related diseases that can make our pets uncomfortable, sluggish, and downright sick. Since pets can't tell us when they are not feeling well, it is important to recognize the signs of sickness before the animal becomes debilitated. Let's look at some early warning signs of serious ailments that older pets are prone to.

Difficulty climbing stairs, difficulty jumping up, tremors/shaking, stiffness or limping can all be signs that a pet is suffering from painful arthritis or possibly a chronic back condition. Sometimes cancer or even kidney failure can cause pain, resulting in these symptoms.

Loss of housetraining, change in litter box habits (cats), increased thirst, and increased urination are common symptoms of diabetes mellitus (sugar diabetes) and kidney failure. Sometimes hormonal imbalances such as Cushing's disease and hypothyroidism will first appear with these symptoms as well.

If your pet experiences a change in activity level, excessive panting, circling/repetitive movements, confusion or disorientation, a change in sleep patterns, excessive barking/meowing, less interaction with family/hiding, and/or decreased responsiveness, he may be suffering from cognitive dysfunction disorder, similar to Alzheimer's disease in people.

Skin and hair coat changes often accompany hormone imbalance or cancer, while coughing, excessive panting, and exercise intolerance could mean heart failure. Lumps and bumps are usually tumors or cysts. Often these are benign, but some swellings are malignant and life threatening.

An increase in appetite accompanied by weight loss in an older cat is a typical sign of an overactive thyroid or hyperthyroidism. Weight gain in older pets is very common and is never healthy. Studies have shown conclusively that animals that maintain a normal weight live longer.

Of course, we also have the ever-popular halitosis or bad breath. Halitosis is usually a sign of periodontal disease or gingivitis. This bacterial infection of the gums is caused by excessive tartar on the teeth and can cause life-threatening internal infections.

If you notice any of the above symptoms in your pet, have him seen by your veterinarian for a full workup. Modern veterinary medicine has much to offer our older pets. There is no longer a need to ignore the pain they are experiencing or to brush their suffering off as simply aging changes.

Also, do not be talked into the latest medications. Consult a holistic veterinarian and consider acupuncture, herbs, and other natural treatments to aid the healing process. Many senior pets benefit from these gentle methods.

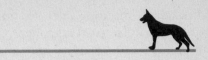

Senior Diseases

Let us look more specifically at some of the diseases common to older animals. Osteoarthritis is an inflammation of one or more joints of the body causing pain and stiffness. In older pets, it is usually caused by years of wear and tear, although the process is accelerated by joint injuries or joint malformations (as with the hip joints in hip dysplasia).

Even if your pet does not whine or cry, you can be sure that arthritis is painful—just ask any person with the condition. There is no reason that a pet would favor a limb other than pain.

It is necessary to take X–rays to tell arthritis from other conditions causing lameness, such as fractures, bone tumors, spinal problems, nerve injuries, and ligament/tendon tears.

There are many anti–inflammatory medications available to help ease the pain and swelling of this disease. There are also natural supplements, such as glucosamine and chondroitin sulphates, that can aid the healing process of the joints. Acupuncture, as well as certain herbal remedies, is also very helpful in the treatment of arthritis. In general, osteoarthritis is a chronic condition requiring life–long treatment.

Studies show that more than half of the senior dogs will die of some form of cancer. This dreaded disease can affect any part of the body, including the internal organs. Exposure to 2–4D weed killer was reported by the National Cancer Institute to induce lymphatic cancer in dogs. Certain vaccines can cause a specific cancer in cats. No doubt, many factors play a roll in the development of malignancy in pets.

Signs of cancer tend to creep up slowly. The symptoms may be obvious, such as a lump on the skin, or other times there may be less specific signs such as weakness or vomiting. Some forms of cancer can be difficult to diagnose, but one thing is certain, the sooner it is detected, the better the prognosis.

It is often necessary to run blood work, X–rays, and a battery of tests to detect internal forms of cancer. Skin tumors can often be diagnosed by needle aspirate (inserting a needle and drawing off cells). This can be done right in the office as an outpatient. Other times it is necessary that the entire tumor, and a wide margin around it, be removed surgically under anesthesia just to diagnose the type.

Treatment of cancer depends on the tumor type. Many times, simply removing the tumor is curative. For malignant tumors, however, other treatments may be needed. Cancer therapy in pets has come a long way in the past twenty years. Chemotherapy can be expensive and cause side effects. Some pets do benefit, but these extreme measures are not for everyone. There are natural treatments, such as homeopathy, herbs, and acupuncture that have been shown to help as well.

Chronic renal failure (CRF) is a very common disease of older dogs and cats. The first signs of kidney failure are increased thirst, increased urine output, decreased appetite, and weight loss. As the disease progresses, there may be vomiting, diarrhea, emaciation, weakness, anemia, seizures, and death.

The diagnosis of kidney failure is based on blood tests, urinalysis, and X-rays. Once diagnosed, special prescription diets are available that are low in protein, which eases the burden on the kidneys. Preparing a special homemade diet is also beneficial.

Renal failure can cause dehydration, and dehydration damages the kidneys, so it is important that the pet has adequate fluid intake. Often it is necessary to hospitalize the pet and give intravenous fluids to correct this problem. Sometimes the pet can be given fluids under the skin as needed on an outpatient basis. I have found acupuncture and herbs to be especially helpful in such cases.

CRF is a progressive, incurable disease. The best we can hope to do is slow its progress and help the animal cope with the symptoms. Even with aggressive treatment, the disease may progress quickly or it can sometimes be managed for years. The key is early intervention, constant owner monitoring, and frequent veterinary follow-up, including blood work and fluids when needed.

Reggie Peterson was a spunky Yorkie I got to know well over the years. At the age of twelve he began drinking excessively and became sluggish. Tests showed that he had developed chronic renal failure. We treated him conventionally with a special kidney diet and gave him fluids as needed to help him.

Gradually, over the course of a few months, his condition became worse and the fluids no longer perked him up. One day his caregivers brought him in requesting euthanasia. I had just started the acupuncture certification course and as I was leaving the room to draw up the fatal injection the thought struck me to offer acupuncture.

Now, my office is in a small town, and the Petersons seemed to be conservative individuals. They had never shown any interest in holistic therapies, and I thought I might get the usual skeptical disapproval I had often gotten nine years ago when I approached conventional people with complementary medical options. To be honest, as a fledgling acupuncturist, I was not always confident in what to expect from the treatments.

Out of concern for Reggie I risked the embarrassment of rejection and as I was half way out of the exam room door I turned back and said, "Hey, there's one thing we haven't tried yet. Would you be willing to have me try acupuncture on Reggie? I'll do the first treatment at no charge, so you have nothing to lose. If it doesn't help, we can put him to sleep later."

To my delight, Reggie's owners were relieved to have another option, as far-fetched as it seemed to them. I treated four points for his kidneys, gave him another injection of fluids for good measure and sent them on their way.

Several days passed without a call from the Petersons. When a week passed with no word, I thought that Reggie might have passed away at home. I called the Petersons and to my surprise they reported that Reggie was eating and playing like his old self.

Periodic acupuncture treatments kept Reggie feeling good for another year and a half. Finally, the Petersons were forced to make the dreaded decision for euthanasia, but they did it knowing they had given him every option and had benefited by having more time with their little friend.

The term "endocrine disorders" refers to a number of diseases that affect the hormone secreting organs of the body. A very common endocrine disorder of older dogs and cats is diabetes. Diabetes mellitus (sugar diabetes) is a condition involving an excess of glucose (sugar) in the bloodstream. It is due to a lack of the hormone insulin, which is necessary for glucose to enter cells where it is needed for energy.

The first signs of diabetes that most pet owners notice are that the pet drinks and urinates excessively. If left untreated, the condition of the diabetic pet deteriorates, and she may lose weight and become weak. Cataracts may form causing blindness. Diagnosis is made by complete physical exam and blood and urine tests showing above normal glucose levels.

Insulin injections are usually needed to correct the situation. They are generally given once a day, but sometimes twice a day injections are needed. Multiple small meals of a low carbohydrate diet help keep the blood glucose on an even keel. Again, holistic therapies often help this condition. Blood and urine glucose levels need to be monitored frequently to maintain the proper glucose level in the blood.

Hyperthyroidism refers to a condition in which there is an excessive amount of thyroid hormone in the system. It is the most common hormone imbalance in middle–aged and old cats. The hormone overload is usually caused by a benign tumor on the thyroid gland.

The classic symptom picture in cats includes weight loss despite an increase in appetite. The increased appetite is due to a sped–up metabolic rate and increased energy demand. Vomiting and diarrhea are sometimes seen because of overeating. Hyperthyroidism affects the kidneys and can cause the cat to drink and urinate more than normal. The disease also affects the heart and can cause an arrhythmia, hypertension, and even heart failure.

Having mentioned all these symptoms, about 10 percent of cats with hyperthyroidism simply become lethargic, weak, and anorexic. Blood work must be done to diagnose this condition. The best test is the measurement of the thyroid hormone T4.

Conventional treatment of hyperthyroidism is accomplished either by blocking thyroid hormone production with medication, by destruction of diseased tissue with radiation, or by surgical removal of the diseased thyroid gland. Homeopathy or Chinese herbs and acupuncture can be used to rebalance the system. Chiropractic also has been helpful in certain cases. This condition must be diagnosed and treated as soon as possible to avoid serious complications.

Cushing's syndrome is common in older dogs and involves a problem with the adrenal glands. Due to a tumor or pretumor condition, the adrenal glands overproduce the hormone cortisol. Signs of this condition are increased thirst, increased urination, increased appetite, hair loss, dark patches of skin, weight gain, muscle weakness, and pendulous abdomen. If left untreated, the condition can be fatal.

Diagnosing Cushing's syndrome can be very difficult. Even specialized blood tests are not 100 percent accurate. Once diagnosed, medication or holistic treatments can control the problem, but frequent monitoring is needed to manage the disease.

When the End Is Near

It is difficult to know what to do for an ailing, aged animal friend. The course of most degenerative diseases associated with old age is tumultuous. There may be many ups and downs. One day the animal looks like she is about to breathe her last breath and the next she is playing like a kitten. What are we to do as guardians, friends, and caregivers?

The first task is to be sure that the problem has been adequately diagnosed. This requires diagnostic tests. Whether you plan to treat holistically or conventionally, the disease must be diagnosed for the animal to be treated properly.

The next step is to formulate a treatment plan. Every veterinarian has his or her own biases and areas of expertise. If you were to take the same sick pet to ten different veterinarians, you would likely get ten different treatment options. If you are unhappy with the approach offered to you, seek a second opinion. It is imperative that you be comfortable with the care that is given to your animal companion at this critical stage of her life.

Be prepared for an emergency. This concept is always important but especially when you are caring for an older pet whose condition could change suddenly. It seems that serious problems seldom happen during normal business hours. Be sure you know the hours that your veterinary office is open and whether or not there is a doctor on call.

In case of an emergency, do not just rush your pet to your veterinarian. If he's not there, you may have wasted precious time. Keep the number of the local emergency clinic handy and be sure you know how to get there. The time to prepare for an emergency is not while you are in the middle of one.

As a pet's health declines it becomes difficult to know what is best for them. Do we struggle to keep them alive, do we let them pass naturally, or do we help them make the transition humanely. It is at this point that we need to remind ourselves that our animal companions came into our lives for a purpose. When they have fulfilled their mission, they are ready to go.

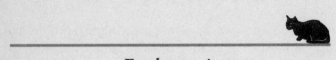

Euthanasia

Euthanasia is a humane way to end an animal's life. The decision to take the life of a beloved pet is often the most difficult choice for a caregiver to make. It is very rare for us to be given such power over the life or death of a loved one. As much as we love our pets, there arise times when difficult decisions must be made.

Euthanasia is a final choice when there are no further options for the pet. It is such a highly charged and personal decision that I always leave it up to the owner. As a veterinarian, I feel it is my place to give the pet owner the prognosis and all treatment options and leave the rest to them.

It is a difficult decision to make for it cannot be taken back. Owners often ask me what I would do if it were my pet. Sometimes the answer is a no-brainer, but often I am compelled to tell the owner that as bleak as the situation may look, sometimes animals surprise even me and recover against all odds.

However, as difficult as it is to take the life of a pet, there are times when euthanasia is the best option. When a patient is suffering from an incurable disease and their quality of life is poor, it is compassionate to end the agony. As stewards of the animal kingdom, we have been given the duty to see to their humane treatment.

Most of us hope that our sickly friend will pass quietly in his sleep, and we will awaken the next morning to find him dead. Unfortunately, it rarely happens that way. For pets, dying a natural death may mean gradually starving to death, or spending their last weeks in excruciating pain.

As pet owners we often grapple with the reason for keeping our pets alive. Are we doing it for the pet or for ourselves? Many times we are haunted by emotions such as guilt and grief. How can we bring ourselves to commission the death of our animal friend? In my view, euthanasia may be the last kind thing a person can do for their pet.

The process of euthanasia is straightforward. A painless injection is given that has the effect of an anesthetic overdose. The animal literally "goes to sleep" and then the heart stops. As simple as this procedure sounds, every veterinarian has his or her own way, and every situation calls for consideration of how to proceed. The tricky thing is that the injection must be given in the vein. For a debilitated, calm pet, this is no problem. However, if the pet is active or has a particularly small vein, the process can be more difficult.

If the euthanasia injection is given out of the vein, it can be painful. It is important that the pet be extremely still. To facilitate this I sometimes give an injection in the muscle that sedates the animal before giving the euthanasia solution.

If you or other family members want to be with your pet during the procedure, be sure to call your veterinarian in advance and be sure of the office policy. Some doctors do not allow the pet owner to be present because of the possible difficulties associated with this emotionally charged event. Occasionally as the pet passes away muscles may twitch, the body may gasp or even vocalize. Sometimes the animal will lose control of the bowels or bladder. It can be very difficult to watch the final breath.

The vast majority of the times the animal closes her eyes and slumps into unconsciousness within seconds of the injection. However, it may take a minute or so for the heart to stop completely.

If she only knew. How difficult it is to say goodbye after all these years. It hurts so badly. I can taste the pain. Guts tied in a knot. I know she can feel it, too.

It seems like just yesterday we were so happy together. We snuggled in the warm sunlight. Playing all our special games. Not a care in the world.

We helped each other through the tough times, too. I couldn't have made it without her. All the memories come flooding back.

But now it is the end. Our paths diverge again. I know it is time to let go. But I can see in her eyes . . . she is not ready to move on. She clings to me, as I cling to her. We are bound together in this painful ball of love and fear.

Why am I holding on to her? Am I being selfish? How can I think of letting her down? How can I end it? What will I do without her?

She knows it is time at last. The final farewell. Cold, dingy rain . . . how fitting. I've done all I can to prepare her.

Oh, the needle. The sweet sting of the needle.

She's crying . . . holding that limp, lifeless body . . . my body. But I'm truly free at last. I'm floating in the sea of love that connects us all . . . forever. What joy! If she only knew.

Making the Decision

When faced with how best to serve your animal friend in the end, it is important to set aside your own needs and desires. Be sure you have your true intention clear in your mind. Focus on your love for your pet and not the fear of his loss. You need to be able to fully let go. Your pet may not be able to move on if held by your longing for him to live.

This is a time when spiritual sources of guidance are most helpful.

Prayer and meditation are especially needed during such situations. Making contact with the divine within can help to keep your intentions on course.

Be aware of your dreams. The creative forces or even the consciousness of your pet may contact you during this altered state. Guidance from dreams can be further enhanced by incubating a dream for guidance. As you are falling asleep, repeat to yourself an affirmation such as, "I will awaken with a dream that will help me understand what to do for Fluffy." Be sure to have your dream journal and pen on your nightstand and use them as soon as you wake up.

Because spiritual guidance requires interpretation, and because your reasoning powers may be biased by the strong emotions surrounding the situation, it is often best to enlist the help of a friend to assist in understanding any messages that come through. Sometimes an impartial third party can clearly see the message that is right in front of our minds more clearly than we can.

This is also a time to practice your skills as an animal communicator. Simply ask your animal companion what you should do. Don't be surprised if you are unable to pick up the answer psychically. Your emotions are likely to block a clear message. However, your pet may answer you in a less subtle way, such as by refusing to eat.

If circumstances call for a quick decision, go with your first instinct, your gut feeling—your intuition. Just gather all the facts and then act.

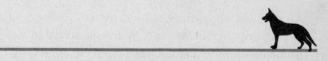

Death

There is something sacred about the moment of death. I have witnessed it many times in my career, as I have eased animals to the other side with the euthanasia injection. I was also blessed by the gift of witnessing my father's last breath. It's not that I've seen the clouds part and a choir of angels singing hallelujah. It is more the realization that at that instant the door to the other side opens to accept another being.

As I have witnessed animals pass, I have often felt a pang in my chest. I originally interpreted this feeling as fear. I imagined the fear that the creature must feel as it leaves the familiarity of its body and loved ones—the fear of the unknown—the fear of death. I am now certain that the fear I felt was more a reflection of my own uncertainties that I projected upon the pet.

Fear is an interesting emotion. It can be quite useful. It can warn us of danger, such as the creepy feeling we may experience when we find ourselves being stared at by a stranger. Fear can call us into evasive action when faced with a dangerous situation. On the other hand, fear can paralyze and debilitate us.

I have heard fear described as "excitement without the breath." Did you ever notice that a fearful feeling is always accompanied by holding your breath? Just breathing deeply during a fearful event can change the feeling of the situation to that of excitement. In fact the Chinese word for fear also means courage.

As I have studied and learned more about my own spiritual nature, I have become less apprehensive about the transition of death. Now, as I put an animal to sleep and I get that familiar pang, I simply breathe through it and feel the excitement that that pet must feel as it moves to the next dimension. I imagine that my breath helps to ease the transition and calm any fears the pet and her human companion may be prone to.

Nugget was a wonderful, spirited Golden Retriever. She had lived a long and happy life with her owner, but at the age of twelve, she developed cancer in one of her lungs. Her caretaker, Nancy, did not want to put Nugget through surgery or chemotherapy, so we decided to keep her comfortable until the cancer got the upper hand.

Two months later, Nugget and Nancy were in my office. The cancer had spread to a lymph node by her shoulder, which had swelled so large that Nugget had a hard time getting around. Even more importantly, Nugget had stopped eating and was no longer enjoying life. Nancy and I knew what we had to do.

There was no need to sedate Nugget since she was a calm dog to begin with and was now further subdued by her disease. I placed the needle in her vein and slowly injected its contents. As the drug started to take effect, Nugget lifted her head, looked Nancy in the eyes and gave a final wag of her tail. I could almost hear Nugget say, "Thank you." Nancy heard it too because at that moment she murmured, "You're welcome."

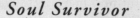

Soul Survivor

Death of the body is inevitable, but life goes on. Death is not the end. Our animal friends help us to affirm this truth. Our lives are forever changed for having known them, and they live on in our memories as we recount their unique contributions in our lives. Some pets live on in even more magical ways.

Fanny was a very special Himalayan cat to Harry and his wife Erma. When Fanny died, the couple had a plan to "bring her back." You see Harry and Erma had a deep belief in the reincarnation of animals. They believed that the energy and intentions of the family could influence the soul elements of the creature in the spirit plane.

The family devised a system using prayer, imagery, and meditation with the intention of holding the consciousness of their beloved feline together and having it reappear in their lives. Following Tibetan tradition on death and soul develop-ment, the family went through their spiritual exercises for forty days.

At the end of this time, they looked in the newspaper for a new cat. They intuitively chose one, and brought it home. Harry and Erma were not surprised when the new kitty began to display some of the same, unique behaviors of their previous cat. Fanny had returned.

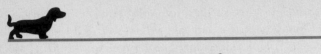

Good Grief

It is easy to understand intellectually that, "There is no death" as Cayce has stated. Many of us have been taught this message in our families and religious communities since birth. A few enlightened individuals even feel this truth in their hearts as they have learned it directly through near–death experiences or other mystical occurrences. Yet, when we lose a loved one, there is no escaping grief. As in touch with the spirit world as anyone may be, there is no denying that we will never experience a dead pet in the same way as when he was alive. We may feel the presence of our beloved friend from time to time, but it is not the same as playing ball or petting him.

Life is full of change. In fact, change is the only constant of our existence. Life is a series of transitions for our pets as well as us. Animals pass from the dependence on their mother in infancy to puppyhood or kittenhood. They develop into adolescence and mature into adulthood. If all goes well, they age into their golden years. Finally, they transition into the sleep of death.

Death is just another phase of the life cycle. Unfortunately, Western culture has forgotten the reality of this statement. We are taught through our media to fight aging with surgery, pills, potions, dyes, and crack fillers. Not long ago we knew enough to honor the wisdom of our elders. Now we discard them. Why the phobia regarding old age? Because it is a reminder of the inevitable next step into the grave.

According to some surveys, the fear of death is eclipsed by the fear of public speaking, but I don't buy it. If such a result is correct, it is only because most people are in such fear of death that they are in total denial. No, death itself is feared most of all. Just look at our human medical practices. Death is seen as our ultimate enemy. It appears to be regarded as preferable to keep a body alive with machinery rather than to admit "defeat." Doctors are often so busy fighting the dragon of death that they forget the compassion needed to prepare the patient and family for the inevitable transition. Thanks to movements such as Hospice that care for the needs of terminal patients and their families, the medical community is beginning to understand the importance of the dying process.

Because our culture fears death, we tend to avoid the grieving process and those going through it. There is a lack of the social supports that used to help mourners. This fact is especially true for those mourning the loss of a pet. There are people in the world who will never understand the bond that many of us share with our pets. Some of these individuals can be cruel with their lack of understanding and compassion. I have seen clients in tears because co-workers have laughed at them for crying over the death of a pet.

> Then we say, when our loved ones, our heart's desires are taken from us, in what are we to believe? This we find is only answered in that which has been given as His promise, that God hath not willed that any soul should perish but hath with every temptation, every trial, every disappointment made a way of escape or for correcting same. It is not a way of justification only, as by faith, but a way to know, to realize that in these disappointments, separations, there comes the assurance that He cares!   1567-2

When a pet dies, a piece of us dies with them. There is a hole in our lives that nothing else can fill. We are wounded by the loss of our companion. Grief is the name given for the healing process involved in becoming whole once again. From this perspective, grief is good.

One never knows how they will handle the death of a pet until they go through it. A person may feel totally prepared for the final farewell, and nevertheless when the news of the passing reaches their ears, there is a bodily, emotional reaction that they may not be ready for. Their world will never be the same without their special friend. Any daily act can remind them of their loss. Not being awakened by that familiar, cold, wet nose on the cheek, the empty spot on the couch where she used to curl up, the cold lap that was always warmed by the furry friend all reinforce the pet's absence.

The loneliness associated with grief can be disorienting. The rest of the world looks normal. Everyone else is going about their business as if nothing is wrong. But for the bereaved everything is wrong. Being out of sync with those around you can add to the loneliness.

Stages of Grief

After a beloved animal passes, her pain is over, but the anguish of the family that she leaves behind is just beginning. Every individual has his or her own way of dealing with loss and everyone needs varying amounts of time to go through the process. At the same time, there are common phases that all seem to share as they grieve. Grief can be a lonely, disorienting experience, so it is important to realize that the feelings a pet lover may be feeling are normal.

The first stage of grief is denial. The physical and emotional jolt caused by the loss can catapult you into a state of numbness and disbelief. Is it true? Is she really gone forever? This isn't happening!

Once, a distraught, older couple burst through the doors to my clinic with the body of their Husky in the arms of the husband. When they put the body on the exam table, it was obvious that the pet had been dead for hours. The eyes were sunken and the body was stiff with rigor mortis. The owners just could not believe it. They insisted that I listen for a heart beat twice before caving into each other's arms in tears.

Anger is often the next emotion to emerge, and it can be expressed in many ways. Anger is sometimes directed outward at those around you. You may feel animosity toward the doctor and hospital staff or you may even attack your family or friends. Even though anger is a natural reaction, it may drive others away, interfering with support when you need it the most. Just as destructively, the anger may be directed inward and cause depression and guilt. When you stop to think about the situation, you may realize that the feeling is out of place, but it just comes out.

The first step in dealing with anger is realizing that it is a normal reaction. You need to face your anger. Hiding it will not make it go away. You'll get through the process more quickly if you take owner- ship of the emotion.

Analyze where the anger is coming from, and assess whether or not you are expressing it appropriately. After you admit the anger to your- self, talk to a trusted friend about how you feel. The sooner you handle the anger, the sooner you can move on through the next stages of grief. Anger is not an emotion to wallow in.

> ... don't get mad and don't cuss a body out mentally or in voice. This brings more poisons than may be created by even taking foods that aren't good.   470-37

Depression can debilitate even the hardiest of individuals. This mood disturbance, cause by anger turned inward, can cause feelings of help- lessness, hopelessness, and powerlessness. The depressed individual tends to withdraw as their ability to experience joy diminishes. Depres- sion may also bring out physical aches and pains, as well as such bodily disturbances as digestive dysfunctions and sleep imbalances.

The feeling of guilt is another effect of internally directed anger. With the assistance of hindsight our inner critics are always ready to chastise us. Of course, hindsight is always 20/20 so there is no outsmarting the inner critic. The question of "what if?" can never be answered. Dwelling on such a mystery will only serve to slow your recovery and sap your energy.

Know in your heart that you did the best you could do with the information you had at the time. No one can expect any more from you. It is simple for me to say, "Forgive yourself." Unfortunately, it is often easier to forgive others than it is to forgive ourselves. If it helps you, ask for forgiveness of God or of your deceased animal companion. Then let the unconditional love of the Creator and the creature flow to you.

Dealing with the emotional turmoil known as the grieving process can bring us to our knees. Hey, while we're down here, why not turn to prayer and meditation. Dialog with the divine within is especially needed during these times of trouble.

At the same time, it is also a good time to turn to the help of our friends. While grieving over a pet, be sure to surround yourself with people who understand the bond you have with your pet. Many cities have pet loss support groups that can be helpful. Ask your veterinarian or local humane society for information on such organizations.

Because emotions are stored in the body, physical as well as energy therapies can assist you in working through your grief. Simple, physical exercise is often useful in the process of release. It can aid your progress to concentrate on your body instead of your emotional state.

Cayce often recommended walking, especially outdoors in nature, as a helpful exercise for any body. Deep bodywork and massage can also be of benefit. Bach flower essences are especially valuable when dealing with emotional issues. Don't forget aromatherapy and homeopathy. Choose whichever of these modalities resonates with you and with the assistance of the appropriate practitioner, deal with the issues that have come up for you.

The grieving process can cause great stress to the body and mind. Be sure to feed your body a healthy diet. This is an especially good time to consider taking extra vitamins and supplements. Also, feed your mind with healthy thoughts. Watch your self–talk closely. Using an affirmation, such as "Every day I'm feeling better and better," may be helpful. Another useful practice for such times of trouble is to simply list the things in your life that you are thankful for each night as you fall asleep.

The Cayce readings affirm that there is only one force, one energy in all of creation. Realize that the energy you are spending feeling angry, depressed, or guilty could be channeled toward something more worth–while. Find something good to do with the energy raised in the grieving process. Champion a cause or help someone else.

> More individuals become so anxious about their own troubles, and yet helping others is the best way to rid yourself of your own troubles. For what is the pattern? He gave up Heaven and entered physical being that ye might have access to the Father.   5081-1

Grief itself is part of life. There is no getting around it, when faced with a loss, we must go through the grief. The challenge is to face the emotions as they come up. Honor the feelings and let them flow through you.

The death of a pet may bring to the surface of your consciousness other related losses that you may not have fully dealt with. If so, then now is the time to deal with them. Consider life as a learning process and the events of your life as teachers. What did you learn from this one?

> For many an individual entity those things that are of sorrow are the greater helps for unfoldment . . .   3209-2

After an animal companion passes on, the caregivers are left with an empty heart and an empty house. Some people swear to me as they leave the office that they will never have another pet—the heartache is too much to bear. Of course, many of those animal lovers end up back at my office in a few weeks with a new pet.

Everyone grieves differently and no one rule applies to all mourning animal lovers; however, I discourage people from going out and getting a new puppy or kitten right after the loss of a beloved animal friend. I think it is important for most people to thoroughly complete the grieving process before entering a new animal relationship. Any grief that is left unprocessed will resurface sooner or later.

Also, if the caregiver has not completely gotten over the loss of the departed pet, the new companion will probably never live up to the expectations. This situation can make getting to really know and train a new pet very difficult. At the same time, in some cases a new animal companion seems to ease the grieving process with their healing presence. Once again, you must decide what is best for you. Just be aware of the importance of the grieving process and explore your motivation for getting a new pet.

Grieving Children

Sometimes we get caught up in our own drama to the point that we forget what the children in the family may be going through. Children can be profoundly affected by the death of an animal friend. Even though it may appear that they have moved on to their next adventure, be aware that they may still be processing the loss and need your support.

Resist the temptation to spare the feelings of your small loved ones by lying to them. This is a mistake. Whatever the circumstances are for the loss of the pet, be up front with the kids. Discuss with them, at the level they are able to understand, exactly what has happened. As much as possible let them participate in the process.

The old story about "Rover" going to live on a farm in the country is as unhealthy for the children as it is for you. Without a doubt, the youngsters will pick up on your true emotions. Your duplicity will only serve to confuse the children. Besides, you will have missed the opportunity to teach the youngsters about death and how it is an inevitable part of life. Learning this lesson in a healthy way and at an early age, will help them deal with the deaths of loved ones as they get older.

For the sake of the family and yourself, consider having some sort of memorial ritual. Such a ceremony can be very meaningful and helpful, especially if you have children. You may want to mimic the burial process of your particular religion, complete with scripture readings. Again, involve the children in the process as much as possible. It is important for the entire family to have closure to aid the grieving process.

Grieving Pets

Animals that live together often form close bonds. They lie together, play together even bicker like an old married couple at times. Just as in close human relationships, an interdependence develops between pets. Since companion animals suffer from a lot of the same emotional upsets that people do, when one member of the "family" passes on, the others are left missing their buddy.

In fact, animals often mirror their owners. If you are grieving over the loss of a pet, you project that energy into your home environment. Be aware that the animals in the household are picking up that energy, which further complicates their condition.

Pets sometimes need help dealing with their grief. I am often asked if the body of the deceased pet should be brought home to be viewed by the surviving animal friends. I think that in some cases this helps, but animals are actually more in tune with what is going on than we give them credit for. On an intuitive level, they know their comrade has moved on. Seeing the body may make the concept more real to them, but I don't think it is usually necessary. You need to use your intuition to make this call. Chances are that if you feel it is important, your animal companions will, too.

So, how else do you help a grieving pet? Do the same things you would do to help a grieving friend. Mostly be there for your pet. Talk to them about how you are feeling. Comfort them, reassure them, and play with them. Make them a part of any memorial service the family creates. You will probably notice that as you work with your companions and they work with you, everyone will start to feel better.

At times, I have seen surviving pets become sick with grief. I don't know if they go through all the same stages that we do, but they definitely get depressed. Some pets become sluggish and refuse to eat for days or even longer. Depression can be dangerous for pets.

You can help them with your support, but do not overlook the possibility of a real physical problem with your pet. The stress of grief can draw out an underlying condition. Any behavior change may be a sign of a medical condition that requires treatment. If your pet is having problems, be sure to have him checked. Also consider the holistic therapies that have helped you deal with your grief. Whatever you find helpful will likely help your animal friend.

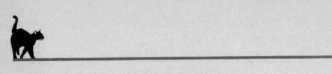

Acceptance

The final stage of the grieving process is acceptance. As we travel the road of mourning at our own pace and in our own ways, gradually the darkness lifts and each day becomes brighter. Acceptance does not mean that we have forgotten our special relationship. It simply means that we can think of our deceased loved one without an overwhelming feeling of sadness. We have learned from the experience of having related with our companion animal. Our life will forever be colored by the love we have shared as we reflect on the lessons that give meaning to our lives.

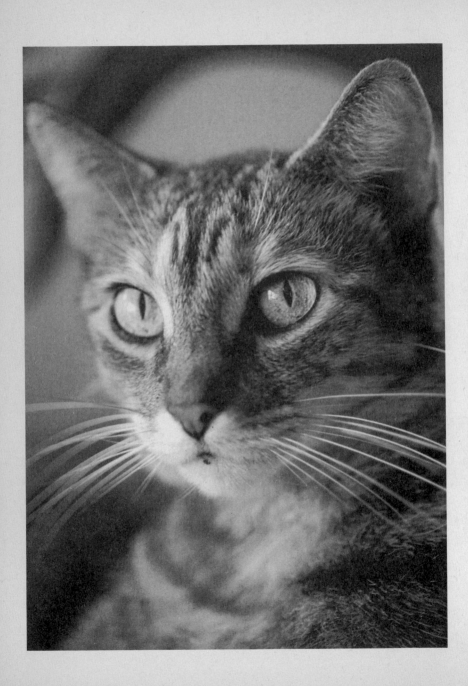

CHAPTER

7

BEYOND

Meditate, oft. Separate thyself for a season from the cares of the world. Get close to nature and *learn* from the lowliest of that which manifests in nature, in the earth; in the birds, in the trees, in the grass, in the flowers, in the bees; that the life of each is a manifesting, is a song of glory to its Maker. And do thou *likewise!*

1089-3

The Edgar Cayce readings often suggested that we should look to nature and the natural world for spiritual guidance. Our ani-mal friends are an extension of that natural world. Humankind has surrounded itself with small keepsakes of nature. We have gathered in the creatures from the cold and rain to care for them as they care for us. We have handcrafted these wild creatures, molding them into helpmates and companions.

Pet Teachers

Why have we chosen to share our lives so intimately with animals? Why do we feel a need to cohabit with other living beings? Perhaps we sense that they hold a key to the great mysteries of existence.

> Go to the ant, thou sluggard—understand his ways and be wise! Remember, of course, the song of the grasshopper, as well as the ant or the bee—but know in Whom ye have believed. For He, the Giver of all good and perfect gifts, has given these—the handiwork of His creation—as a pattern or example or lesson, that ye—too—may learn.   1965-1

Apparently even the lowly ant has something to teach us. Other living beings have been provided for us not as entertainment or as beasts of burden, but rather as a "pattern or example or lesson." Nature and animals are our teachers in the classroom of life.

So just what are we to learn from the experience of sharing our lives with our furry companions? What is gained from the pet connection? The lessons are many. In fact, I would venture to say that the lessons we gain from our relationships with the animal kingdom are as numerous and unique as the many animal connections that exist.

Our animal companions are a reflection of ourselves. It is amazing to me how many people so closely resemble their animal companions, not just physically but mentally and emotionally as well. The Cayce readings concur that our relationships offer an opportunity for self-exploration.

> For constantly is the soul-entity meeting self in its activities, in its relationships.   1604-1

I believe that every pet connection qualifies as such a relationship that allows us to see ourselves more clearly. If there is something about your pet that really annoys you, then that may be telling you something about yourself. If there is a quality of your pet that you are inspired by, then look closely at that as well.

Furthermore, as we truly relate with our pets and come to know ourselves, we can learn our true calling as individuals.

> Man ... is in that position where he may gain the greater lesson from nature, and the creatures in the natural world; they each fulfilling their purpose, singing their song, filling the air with their perfume, that they—too—may honor and praise their Creator; though in their humble way in comparison to some, they each in their *own* humble way are fulfilling that for which they were called into being, reflecting—as each soul, as each man and each woman should do in their particular sphere—*their* concept of their Maker!
>
> 1391-1

The animals in our lives are a reminder that we each have a unique purpose for being alive. Each individual has a matchless concept of their Maker to reflect. If we join wholeheartedly in the process of sharing life with our pets, we may be inspired to reach our full potential.

Inspiration

One quality of companion animals that always touches me as a healer is simply their ability to inspire those around them.

Richie is an elderly tabby cat with a lot of attitude. I met him on a chilly January morning and knew immediately that we were dealing with a serious situation. He had been diagnosed six months earlier by his regular veterinarian with a malignant nasal tumor and had been given a grave prognosis. By this time the tumor had eaten its way through his skull and produced a large mass between his eyes.

In spite of his disfigurement, Doreen, his caregiver, was not ready to give up. He was eating well and enjoying life. Doreen felt that he still had something to offer, some purpose to live for. She brought him to me looking for alternatives that might give him comfort as the cancer progressed. I started him on herbs and acupuncture treatments.

Over the months Richie's tumor slowly grew larger but he happily maintained his routine. By June, however, he was starting to have problems. The malignant growth was beginning to engulf his right eye and his appetite was waning. One night he had a terrible nose bleed. Doreen rushed him to an emergency hospital. The doctor urged Doreen to consider euthanasia, but a look and a nudge from Richie indicated it was not his time yet.

By the time I saw him a few days later, Richie looked like he was nearing the end. He had not eaten a bite for a week and had lost his spry attitude. After a heart-to-heart discussion, Doreen decided to give him one more acupuncture treatment and then take him home. He was now over seventeen years old and had had a long, happy life. She wanted him to pass away in familiar surroundings.

I changed my acupuncture treatment approach. Instead of points to fight the cancer, I used a combination that would decrease pain and help him attune to the Cosmos to ease his impending transition. However, within a couple of days, instead of his health declining, Richie's appetite began to return. Doreen sought the counsel of a local animal communicator who explained to the ailing cat about the tumor and the treatments. Richie's attitude brightened further. He finally understood what was going on with him.

A week later, I saw Richie and was pleased that he was eating well. After the acupuncture treatment, he had a second session with the animal communicator. This time Doreen asked the intuitive if Richie could be instructed on how to visualize the shrinking of his tumor. According the animal communicator, he was willing to try. Doreen, Richie, and the communicator worked together on this visualization causing a noticeable change in his attitude.

The next week when Doreen brought Richie into the treatment room I was stunned by what I saw. His malignant tumor was getting smaller. I continued the acupuncture treatment and two weeks later the tumor was gone. My staff and I could not believe our eyes. He was left with a large, shallow divot in his forehead where the tumor had eaten away the bone.

How could this possibly happen? Perhaps the acupuncture treatment readjusted his energy to help his body throw off the dreaded disease. Maybe by aiding his connection to the Divine he was able to channel healing energy to himself.

Possibly the animal communicator and the group visualization sessions did the trick. Or, could it have been Doreen's and my willingness to let go that sparked his revival? No doubt a combination of the above factors caused his remarkable recovery. One thing for sure is that this medical marvel taught everyone who saw it several important lessons: (1) Even with animals healing comes from within, (2) Truly anything is possible, and (3) Never underestimate the power of a determined feline.

Holistic healing requires the participation of all levels of those involved with the patient. With this kind of cooperation there are no limits. As for Richie, he continues to inspire us all with a renewed sense of holistic healing, perhaps fulfilling his purpose.

Animal Attunement

Our animal companions are bridges that link us to the rest of nature, including our own true human nature. As we come to more fully know ourselves through our pet connections, we gain an understanding of our higher natures. Knowing our own higher selves kindles an awareness of God.

> For Life as it manifests, whether in the grass, the rose, the tree, the dog, the cat, the bird, the animal, *is* a manifestation of that ye worship as God.   1367-1

Perhaps instinctively we have joined together with the animals in an attempt to recapture the Garden of Eden—to catch a glimpse of a time when humans, animals, and the Divine shared the world in harmony.

The Cayce readings suggest that relating with animals can help us to attune.

> Hence we find that the experiences of the entity in the country, in those places close to nature, where the rain,

the sea, the sun, the sand, the trees, the birds, the animals
of nature of today may be about the entity, may *attune* the
entity to a greater ability in the bringing to the consciousness of self and others the awareness of *nature* as a teacher
to mankind!   1786-1

When we attune to the lessons from nature and from our pets, we
realize that we are a part of creation and not superior to it. We are one
with both nature and the Divine as the following exchange acknowledges.

(Q) How is the best way to explain God to a child under
twelve years of age?
(A) In nature. As the unfolding of that that is seen *about*
the child itself, whether in the grasses, the flowers, the
birds, or what; for each are an expression of the Creative
Energies in its activity, and the sooner *every soul* would
learn that they themselves are a portion of everything
about same, with the ability within self to make one's self
one *with* that that brought *all* into being, the change is as
that of service in its *naturalness*.   5747-1

I have often heard teachers of meditation advise their students to be
sure to remove animals from the room when meditating. Apparently
the concern is that pets will interfere with the attunement. It is certainly
true that pets seem to be drawn to those in meditation. They appear to
enjoy being around that peaceful energy. However, there is no need for
animal lovers to allow this fellowship to distract them.

I sat in silent meditation, legs crossed, hands loosely folded in my lap. The
couch upon which I sat looks out the picture windows into the woods behind our
home. As the silence took me deeper, there was a stir on the floor to my right.
With a soft thud, I was joined by one of our four cats. He strolled onto my lap
and began nuzzling my hands. His wet nose tickled my fingers. It had to be Blaze
the, blue-eyed, Flame-Point Siamese. He is the only one who would be so—the

word that comes to mind is—obnoxious. He is the youngest of the cats and loves to fool around.

I ignored his caresses. I was certain that my quiet mood would calm him. But Blaze was not to be denied. He began, first pawing then biting at my shirt buttons. A smile played on my lips as I maintained my peaceful awareness. With my eyes still closed, I stroked his head a few times. My hand glided over his sleek fur. He slowly crawled off my lap but soon returned for more.

As he nibbled at my shirt, I again petted his head gently with the intention of sharing the attunement I was experiencing. Using my imagination, I felt the energy leave my palm and enter his body. Within seconds he lay beside me with his head resting on my knee. He purred gently. The soft vibration filled my body. For me, this shared pulsation became a metaphor for our shared life force. I began to experience the oneness of all as I melted into the Spirit.

It is just possible that relating holistically—body, mind, and soul—with our animal friends may offer us a pathway to enlightenment. I am not saying that pets are THE way of coming to know the Divine but only one of many means available to choose from. Certainly it is a path upon which we animal lovers gladly travel.

As we fully engage in our pet connections we come to know our animal companions, ourselves, nature, and God. This special sharing leads to a communion with all life that invigorates our entire being. Our awareness broadens and we are smitten by the feeling of appreciation for the generosity of God's copious bounty. We are inspired to participate wholly in life and give freely of our own unique gifts. When the student is ready, the pet will appear.

Resource List

Dr. Douglas Knueven
Beaver Animal Clinic
357 State Street
Beaver, PA 15009
724–774–8047
Beaveranimalclinic.com

Betsy Crouse www.animalconnections.com

Renee Takacs 412–257–1289

Agnes J. Thomas, Ph.D. www.petstellthetruth.com

Academy of Veterinary Homeopathy (AVH)
P.O. Box 9280
Wilmington, DE 19809
Phone: 866–652–1590
E–mail: office@theavh.org
www.theavh.org

The American Academy of Veterinary Acupuncture (AAVA)
P.O. Box 1532
Longmont, CO 80502–1532
Phone: 303–772–6726
E–mail: office@aava.org
http://aava.org

American Holistic Veterinary Medical Association (AHVMA)
2218 Old Emmorton Road
Bel Air, MD 21015
Phone: 410–569–0795
Fax: 410–569–2346
E–mail: Office@AHVMA.org
www.ahvma.org

American Veterinary Chiropractic Association (AVCA)
    442154 E. 140 Rd.
    Bluejacket, OK 74333
    Phone: 918-784-2231
    Fax: 918-784-2675
    E-mail: AmVetChiro@aol.com
    www.animalchiropractic.org

Complementary and Alternative Veterinary Medicine
    www.altvetmed.com

A.R.E. PRESS

The A.R.E. Press publishes books, videos, and audiotapes meant to improve the quality of our readers' lives—personally, professionally, and spiritually. We hope our products support your endeavors to realize your career potential, to enhance your relationships, to improve your health, and to encourage you to make the changes necessary to live a loving, joyful, and fulfilling life.

For more information or to receive a free catalog, call:

1–800–723–1112

Or write:

A.R.E. Press
215 67th Street
Virginia Beach, VA 23451-2061

BAAR PRODUCTS

A.R.E.'s Official Worldwide Exclusive Supplier of Edgar Cayce Health Care Products

Baar Products, Inc., is the official worldwide exclusive supplier of Edgar Cayce health care products. Baar offers a collection of natural products and remedies drawn from the work of Edgar Cayce, considered by many to be the father of modern holistic medicine.

For a complete listing of Cayce-related products, call:

1–800–269–2502

Or write:

Baar Products, Inc.
P.O. Box 60
Downingtown, PA 19335 U.S.A.

Customer Service and International: 610–873–4591
Fax: 610–873–7945
Web Site: www.baar.com   E-mail: cayce@baar.com

DISCOVER HOW THE EDGAR CAYCE MATERIAL CAN HELP YOU!

The Association for Research and Enlightenment, Inc. (A.R.E.®), was founded in 1931 by Edgar Cayce. Its international headquarters are in Virginia Beach, Virginia, where thousands of visitors come year-round. Many more are helped and inspired by A.R.E's local activities in their own hometowns or by contact via mail (and now the Internet!) with A.R.E. headquarters.

People from all walks of life, all around the world, have discovered meaningful and life-transforming insights in the A.R.E. programs and materials, which focus on such areas as personal spirituality, holistic health, dreams, family life, finding your best vocation, reincarnation, ESP, meditation, and soul growth in small-group settings. Call us today at our toll-free number:

1–800–333–4499

or

Explore our electronic visitors center on the Internet: **http://www.edgarcayce.org.**

We'll be happy to tell you more about how the work of the A.R.E. can help you!

A.R.E.
215 67th Street
Virginia Beach, VA 23451-2061